STUDENT'S EDITION

VICTORYXR PRESENTS

HUMAN ANATOMY

AUGMENTED REALITY (AR)

GUIDE TO THE VITAL ORGANS

Executive Producer
Steve Grubbs

Curriculum Specialist
Rene Gadelha

Science Advisor
Wendy Martin

Development Team
Cody Birks
Aaron Hagens
Tyler Halterman
Sorine Jil
Alec Pilola
Tyler Turner

Publisher
VictoryXR

TABLE OF CONTENTS

MEET YOUR INSTRUCTORS

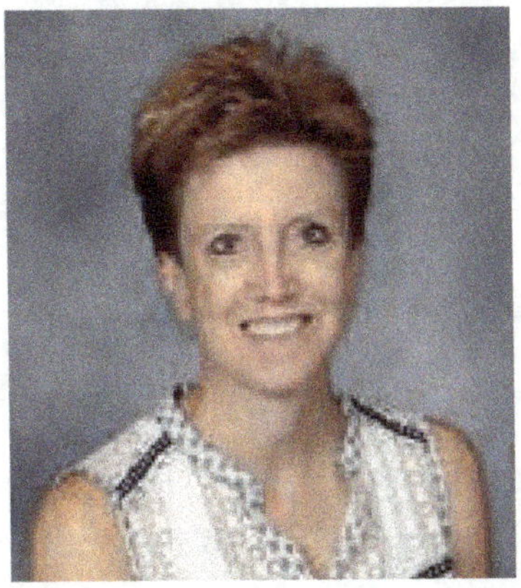

WENDY MARTIN

NATIONALLY-RECOGNIZED SCIENCE TEACHER

Wendy has been teaching high school and college level science classes for more than 20 years. In addition to her teaching role, Wendy also provides guidance as a consultant to many VictoryXR STEM projects. In this secondary role, she writes scripts, researches science data, and serves as the teacher guide in numerous XR videos which are all aligned to Next Generation Science Standards (NGSS).

Earning her Masters Degree in Biology, as well as Education & Technology, Wendy has the broad background necessary to integrate VR and AR in a substantive way into STEM curricula. Wendy is a dynamic educator, full of energy which comes through her facilitation of the lessons. She enjoys creating and delivering material in up-to-date and relevant ways.

Of special note, Wendy received the prestigious local Jaycee Outstanding Young Educator Award in 2006 and was the recipient of the *Live! With Kelly* Top Teacher Award in 2012.

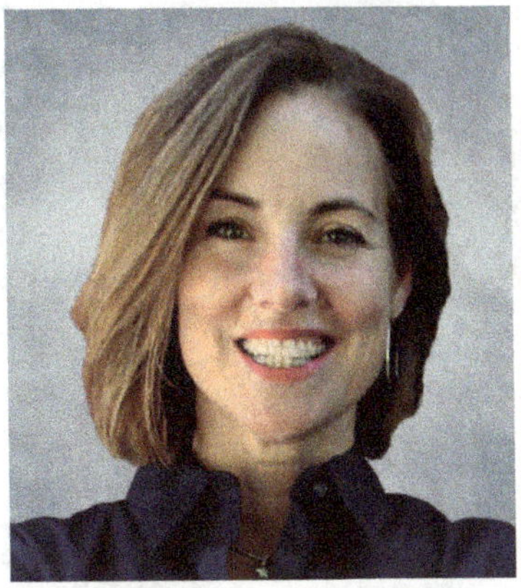

RENE GADELHA

CURRICULUM SPECIALIST

Rene has been deeply involved in education for more than 25 years. Building upon her own studies, including an English undergraduate degree, permanent teaching certification, and a Masters Degree in Instruction & Curriculum, Rene is a leader in the education field. A former classroom teacher, Rene has also been a consultant on educational materials to Pearson Education, College Board, ETS, and CTB-McGraw Hill.

Outside of the classroom, Rene has impacted multiple school districts by serving as a director on two different school boards (Iowa & New Jersey) . Professionally, Rene has been intrigued at the blending of education standards, science concepts, and new technologies and has transitioned into her current role as Vice President of Curriculum at VictoryXR.

Of special note, Rene was appointed to the Iowa Governor's STEM Advisory Council in 2017 and remains an active member.

USER GUIDE

Downloading App Instructions

- Go to the Apple App Store or the Google Play Store and search "AR Lab Book: Vital Organs".
- Download the App.
- Open the App.
- Hover your device over the AR marker on the left side of the page.
- Choose from the various options on your screen to interact with the book.

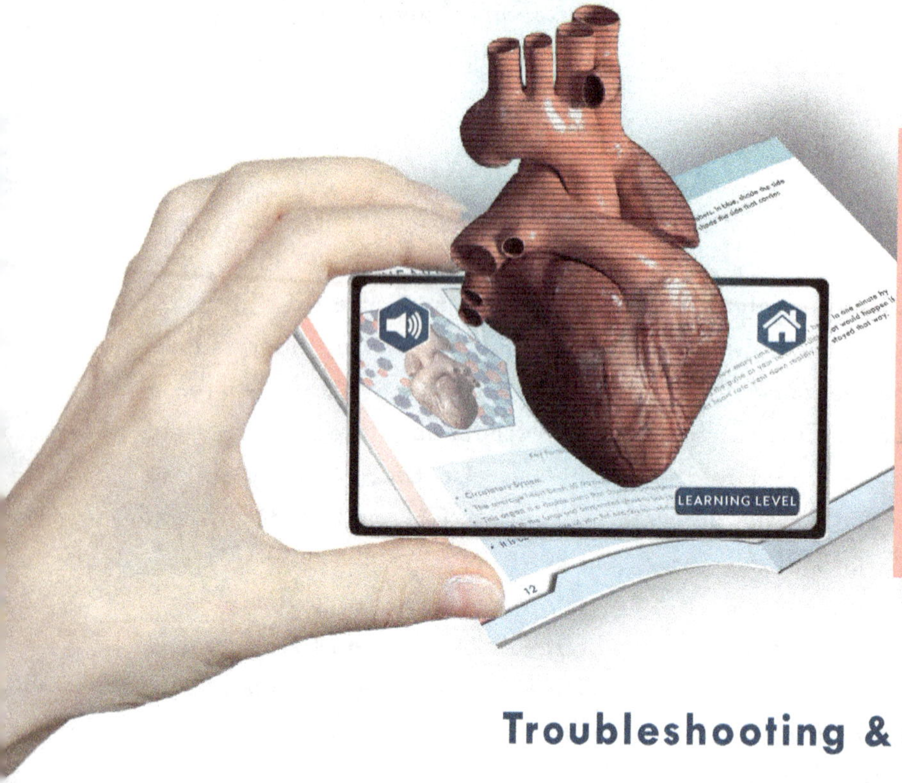

Two audio clips are featured for each **organ**, narrated by award-winning science teacher, Wendy Martin. Clips are approximately 20-30 seconds long, for both ***Basic*** and ***Advanced*** learning levels.

Troubleshooting & Help

VictoryXR.com/ARTroubleshoot

800-670-5716

info@victoryxr.com

VXR.Direct

ENGAGING WITH AR MARKERS

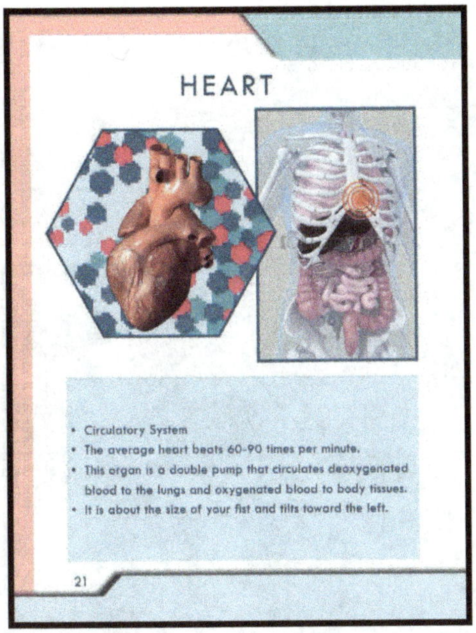

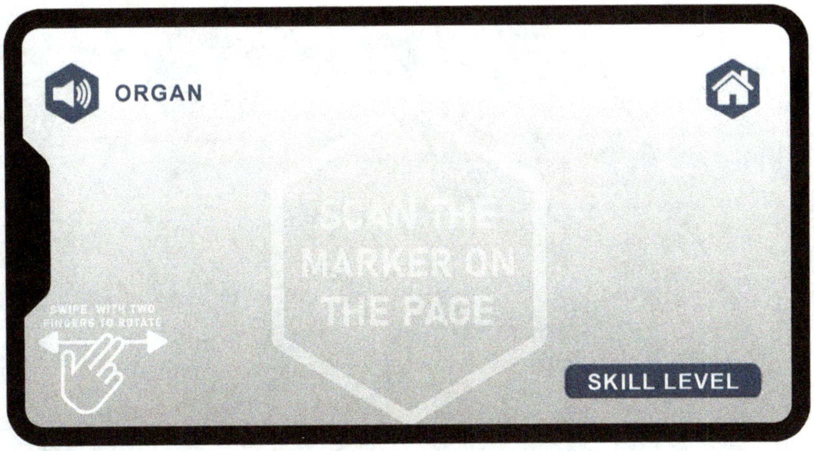

AR markers appear on the left page. They contain an image of an organ atop multi-colored circles.

Hover device over the AR marker to activate and engage an organ in augmented reality.

Tap the speaker icon or the organ title to play or pause the audio clip.

Rotate the organ for multiple views using two fingers and swiping left or right. A pinching motion zooms in and out.

Tap the home icon to return to the main menu.

The bullseye target indicates the specific area where the organ is located inside of the body.

VOCAB WORDS

Bolded words indicate glossary terms, with corresponding phonetic pronunciations located in the back matter.

SKILL LEVEL

Two audio clips are available per organ: ***Basic*** and ***Advanced***. Toggle between them to differentiate learning.

HUMAN BODY (SHELL)

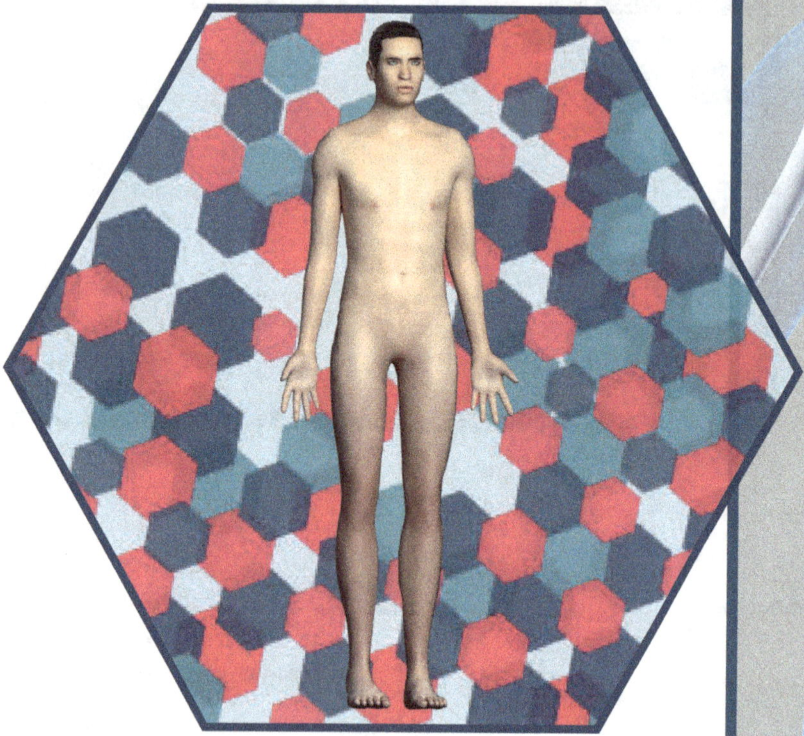

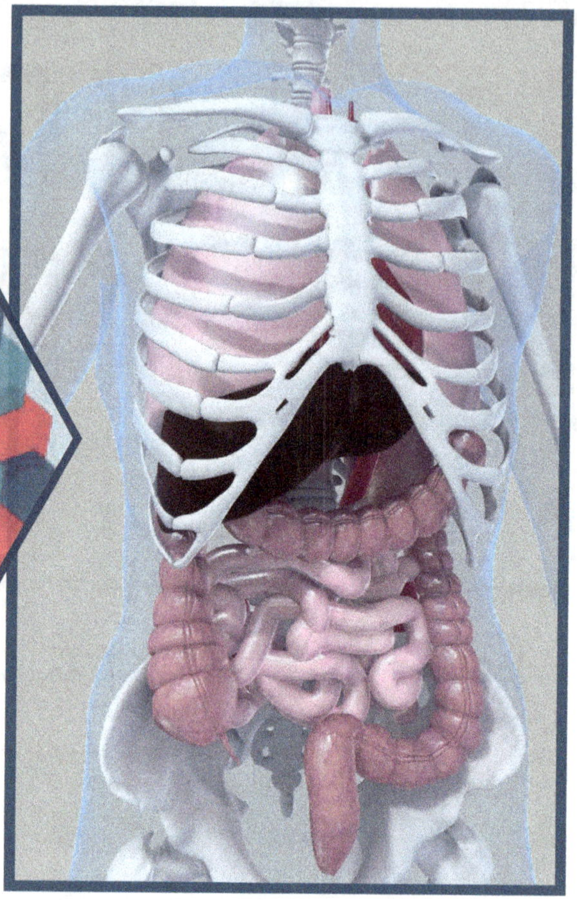

Key Features

- The human body contains 11 different systems.
- Systems are composed of multiple **organs.**
- The systems collectively perform all necessary life functions and maintain **homeostasis.**
- The structure of an **organ** is important to its function.

Play audio to learn more.

Questions & Activities

Provide two examples of how different body systems work together.

Which system do you think is the most important? Why?

HEART

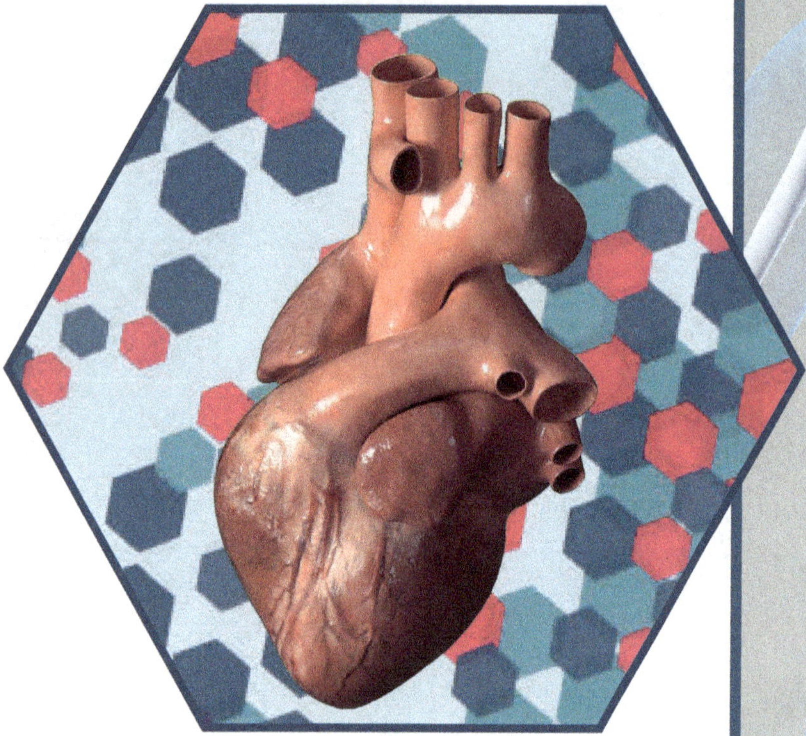

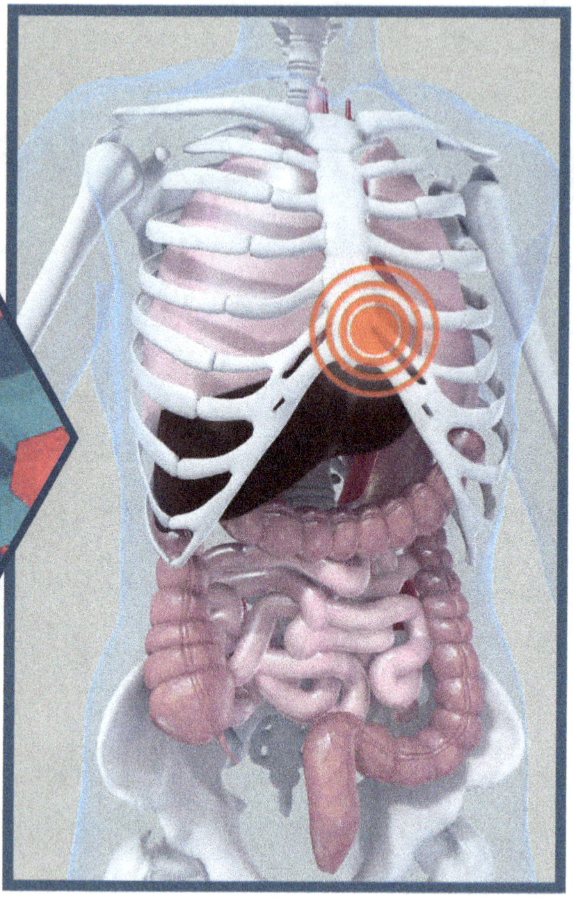

Key Features

- The heart is a vital **organ** of the **circulatory system.**
- The average heart beats 60-90 times per minute.
- This **organ** is a double pump that circulates deoxygenated blood to the lungs and oxygenated blood to body **tissues.**
- It is about the size of your fist and tilts toward the left.

Play audio to learn more.

Questions & Activities

Sketch a heart and label the four chambers. In blue, shade the side that carries deoxygenated blood. In red, shade the side that carries oxygenated blood.

Calculate how many times your heart beats in one minute by taking the pulse at your neck. Predict what would happen if that heart rate went down rapidly and stayed that way.

LUNGS

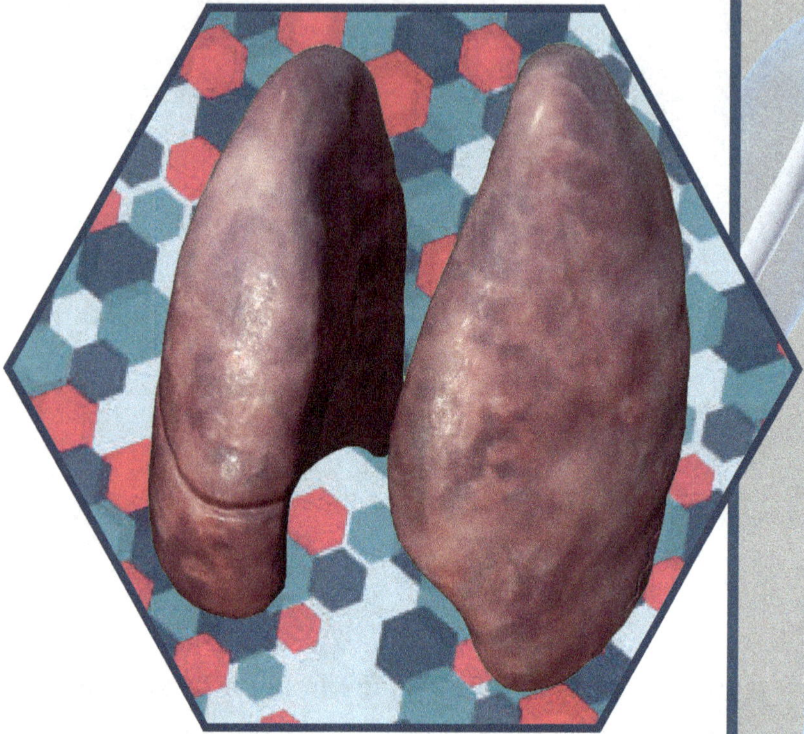

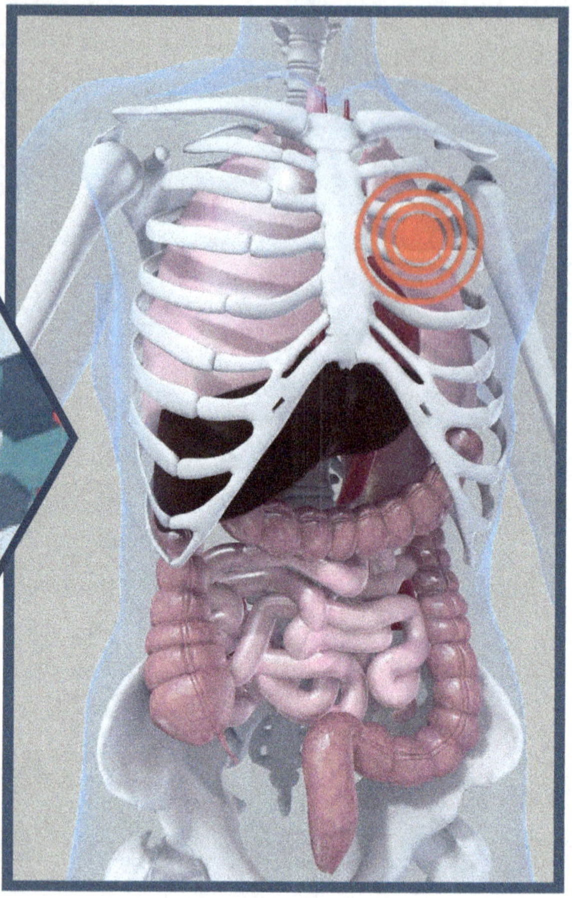

Key Features

- The lungs are a vital **organ** of the **respiratory system.**
- These function as **organs** of gas exchange.
- Oxygen enters the blood for transport and carbon dioxide enters the lungs for exhalation.
- Microscopic **alveoli** are the site of gas exchange within the lungs.
- They can hold approximately 6000ml of air but only move about 500ml in a normal breath.

Play audio to learn more.

Questions & Activities

Name three diseases that involve the lungs.

Identify common symptoms for at least one of the diseases listed above.

DIAPHRAGM

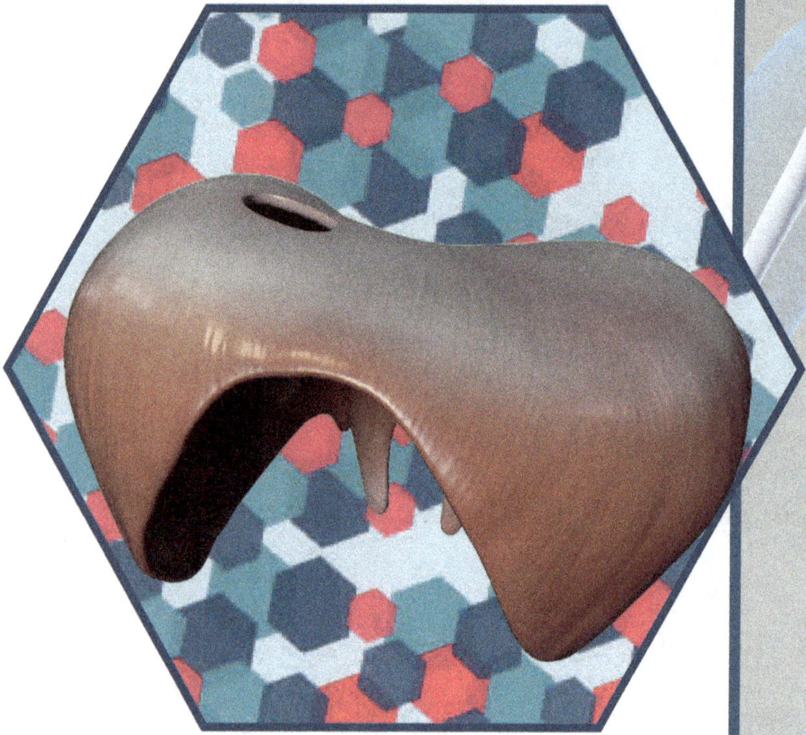

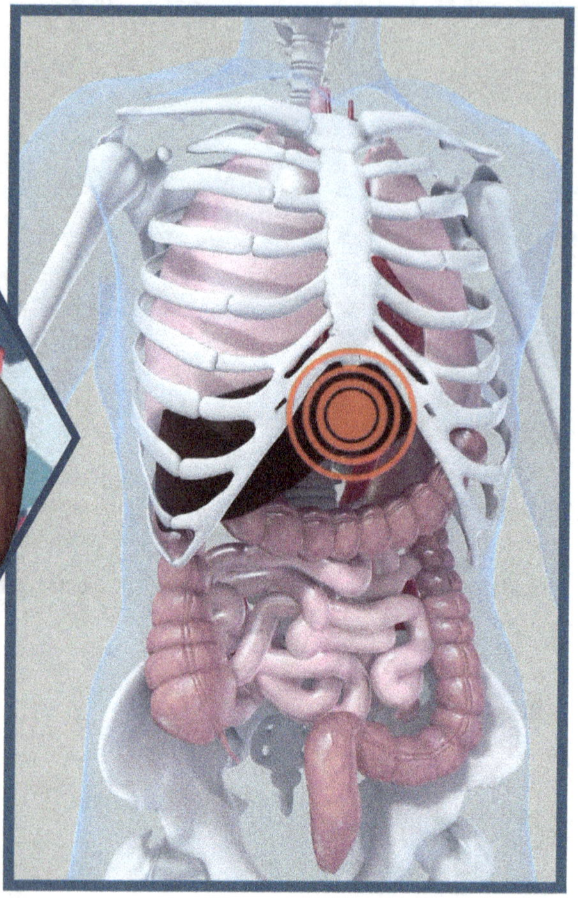

Key Features

- The diaphragm is a vital **organ** of both the **muscular** and **respiratory systems.**
- During inhalation, the diaphragm contracts and moves down; however, during exhalation, it moves back to its resting position.
- It is controlled by the **phrenic nerve.**

Play audio to learn more.

List two systems with **organ**s that pass through the diaphragm.

Which of the three muscle types is the diaphragm classified as: cardiac, skeletal, or smooth? Why?

ESOPHAGUS

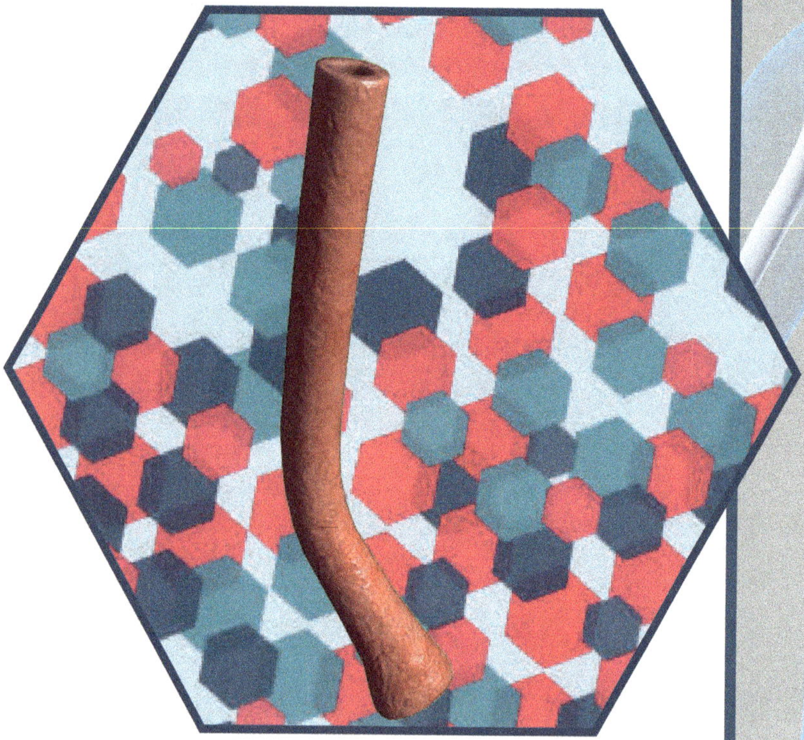

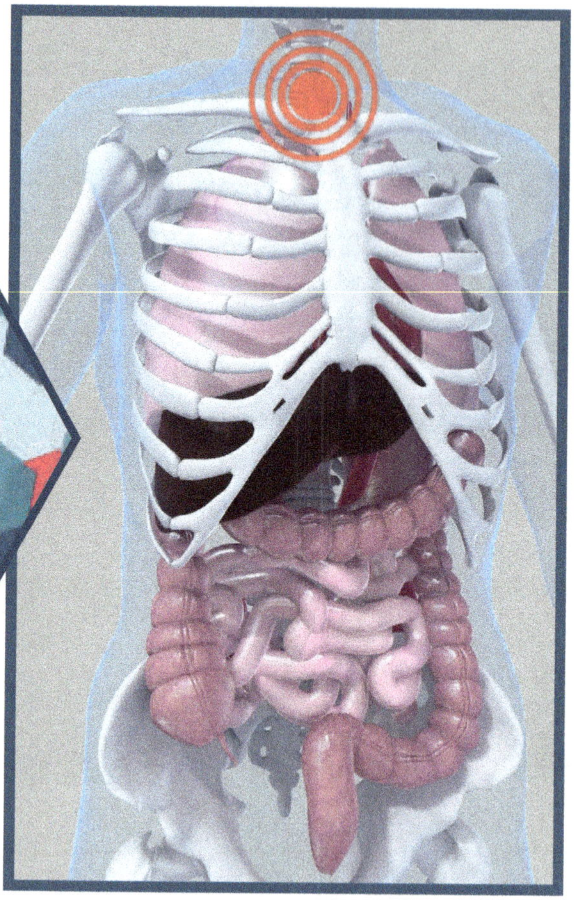

Key Features

- The esophagus is a vital **organ** of the **digestive system.**
- It connects the pharynx to the stomach.
- It has a **sphincter** muscle to prevent backflow of food and fluid.
- The **esophagus** moves food through **peristalsis.**

Play audio to learn more.

What neighboring tube shares the pharynx with the esophagus?

Would the esophagus be affected by acid reflux disease? Explain.

TRACHEA

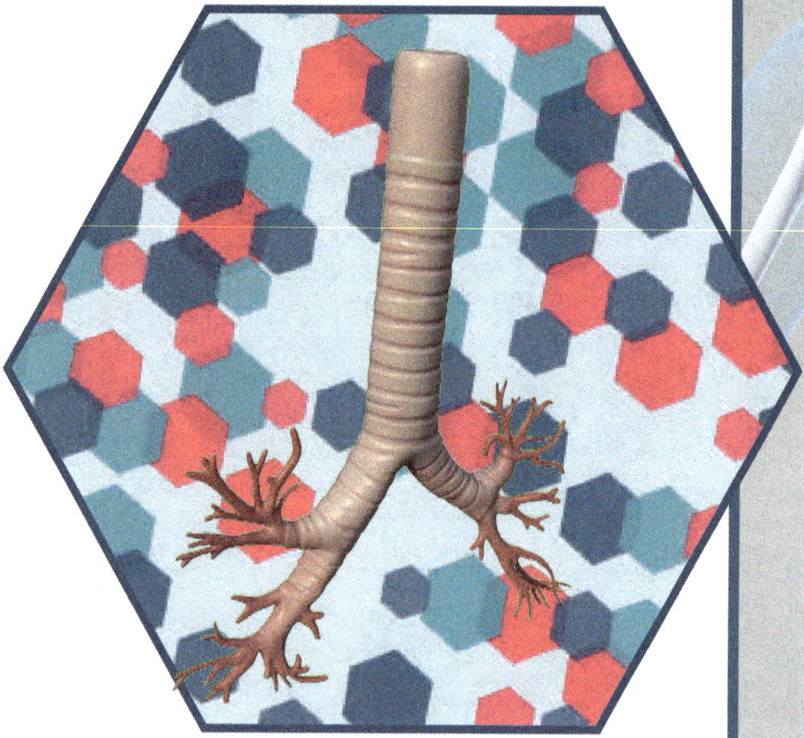

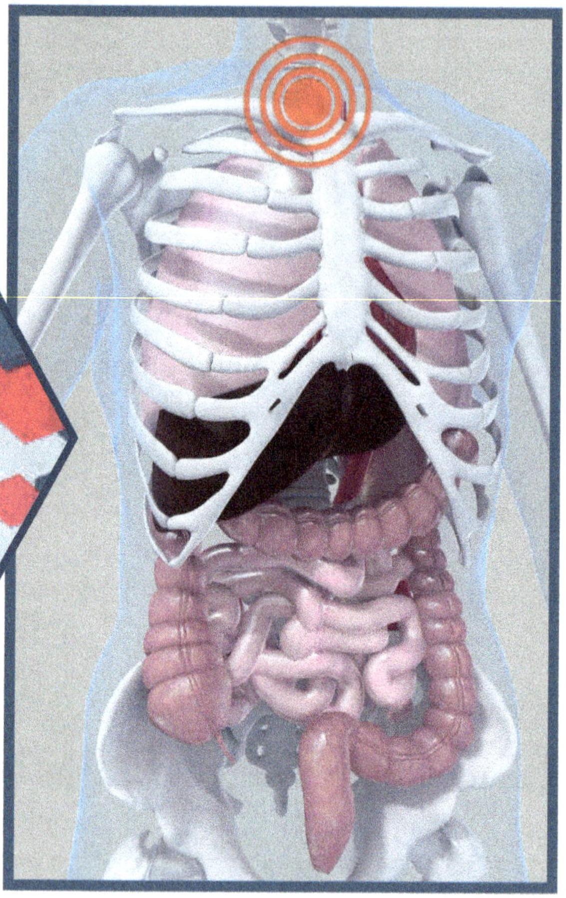

Key Features

- The trachea is a vital **organ** of the **respiratory system.**
- "Windpipe" is another term for this structure.
- It conducts air to and from the lungs.
- C-shaped cartilage rings protect it.
- The **trachea** branches into the bronchi in the lungs.

Play audio to learn more.

What would happen if the **epiglottis** failed to protect the trachea?

What is a tracheotomy?

KIDNEYS

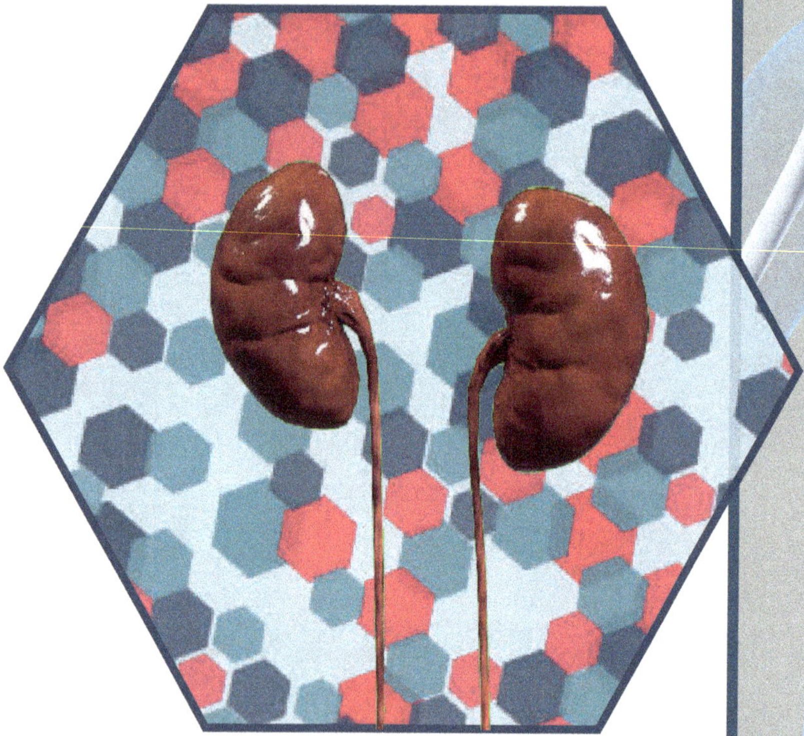

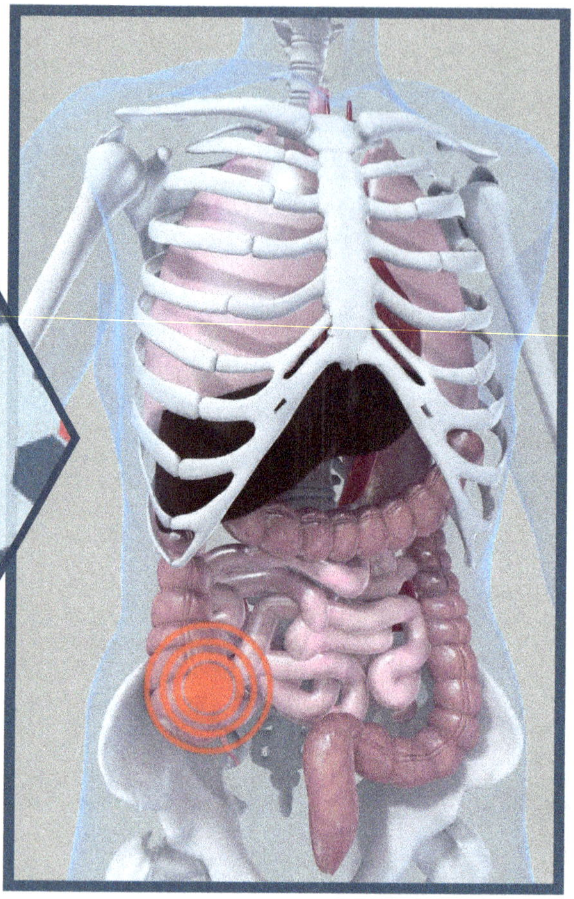

Key Features

- The kidney is a vital **organ** of the **excretory system.**
- The kidneys' main purpose is to filter blood and remove waste and excess ions to form urine.
- The **nephron** is the basic unit of function in a kidney.
- The kidneys also assist in maintaining fluid volumes, pressures, ion concentrations, and pH levels.

Play audio to learn more.

Why would a person need kidney dialysis?

What is a potential health problem for athletes injecting EPO on a regular basis?

STOMACH

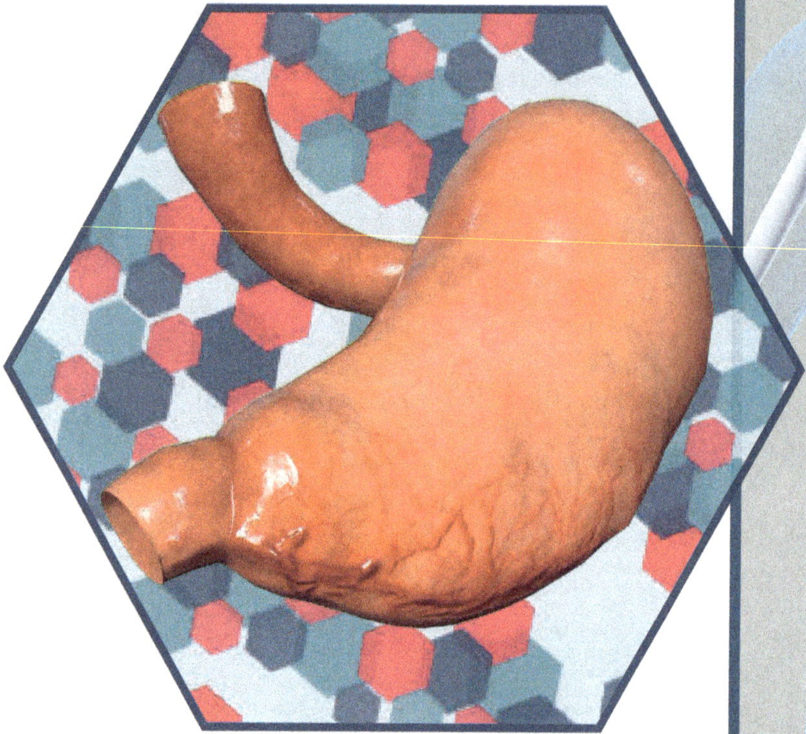

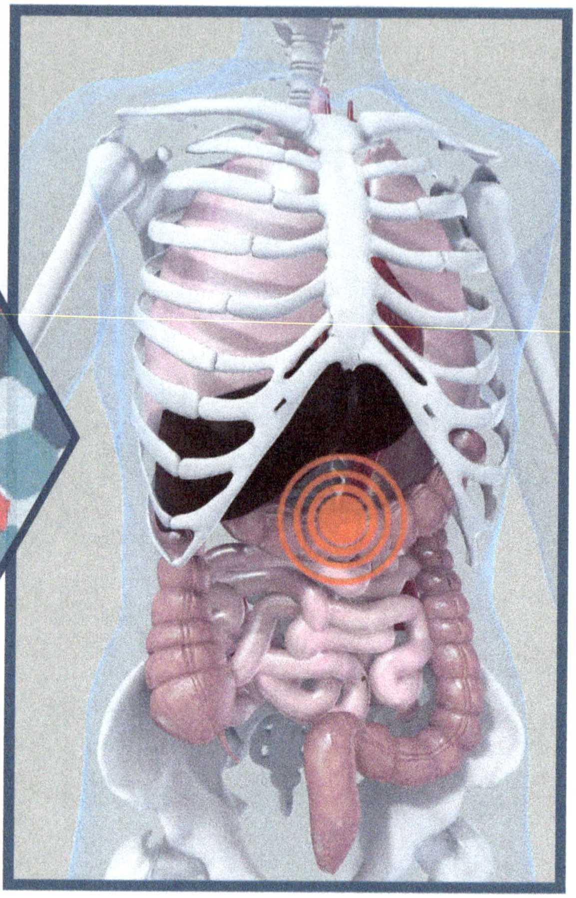

Key Features

- The stomach is a vital **organ** of the **digestive system.**
- It mechanically grinds up food received from the esophagus.
- This **organ** secretes gastric juices that begin chemical digestion of proteins.
- It secretes a coat of mucus to protect itself from the acidity of digestion.

Play audio to learn more.

Questions & Activities

Why is an open stomach wound dangerous to the entire abdominal cavity?

Sketch what a stomach looks like post-gastric bypass surgery.

BLADDER

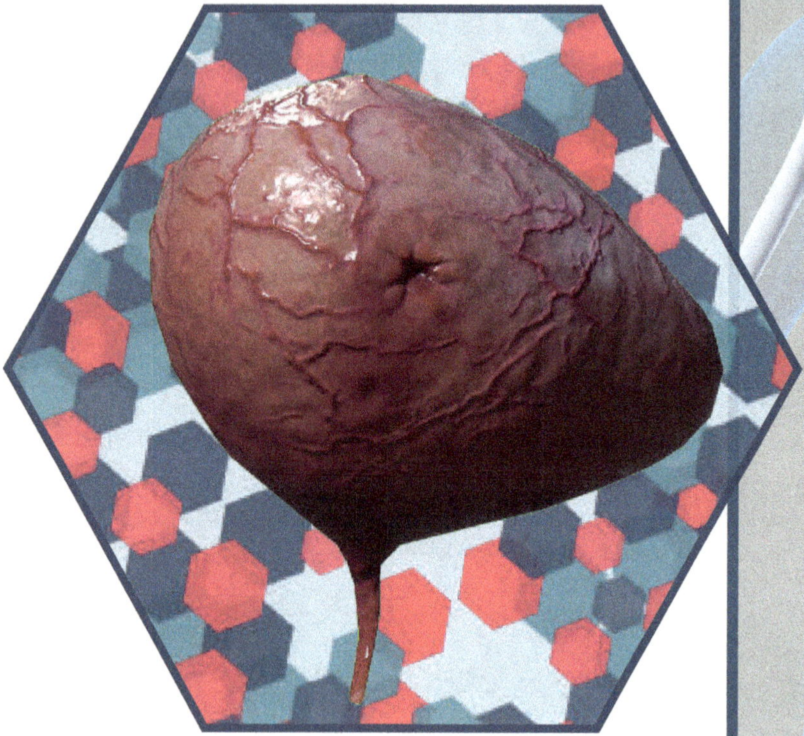

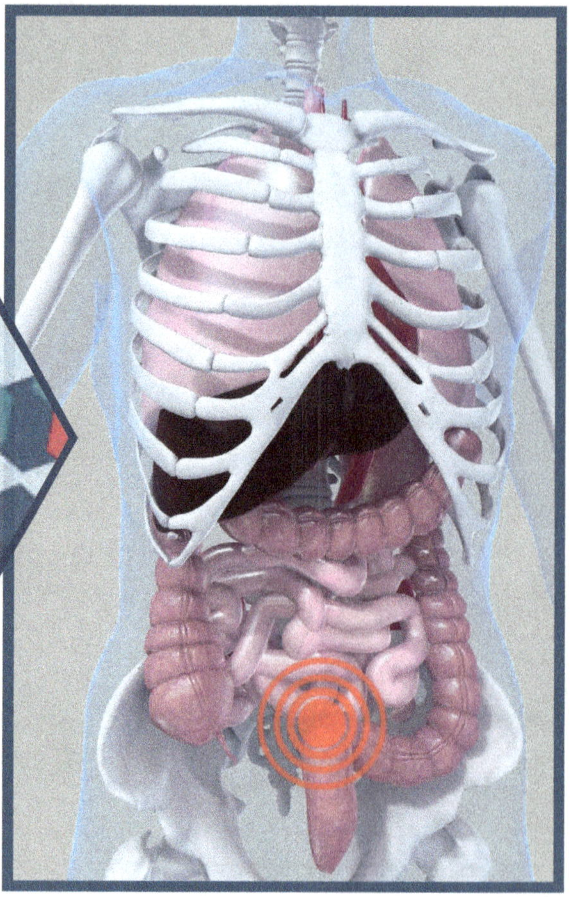

Key Features

- The bladder is a vital **organ** of the **excretory system.**
- This **organ** receives urine from the kidneys.
- It stores urine until disposal by urination through the **sphincter** valves.
- A muscular, expandable **organ,** the bladder can hold up to 1000ml of urine.

Play audio to learn more.

How would the enlargement of the male prostate gland affect urination?

What is unique about the bladder's epithelial tissue?

SKIN

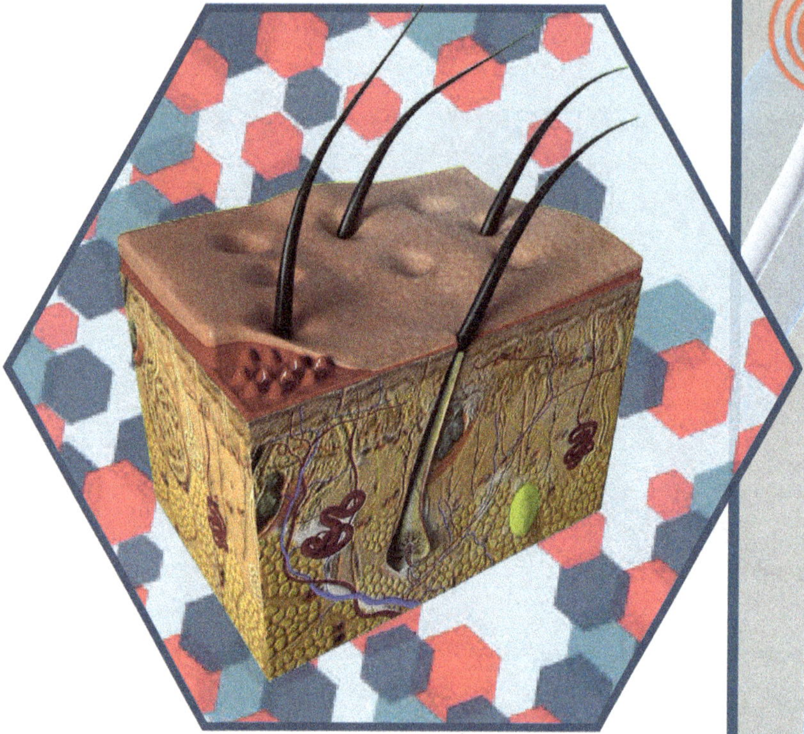

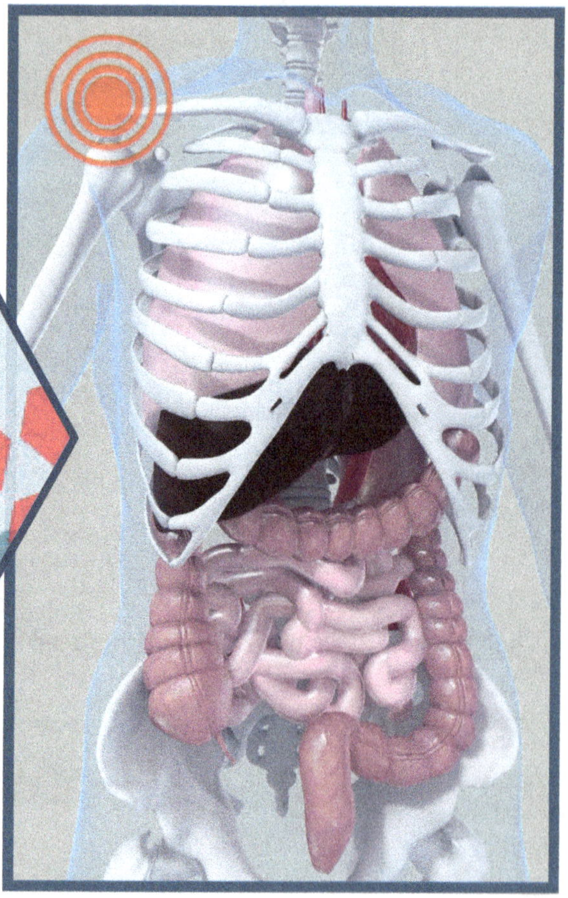

Key Features

- The skin is a vital **organ** of the **integumentary system.**
- It is the largest **organ** of the human body, measuring more than two square meters.
- Three layers comprise the skin: **epidermis, dermis,** and **subcutaneous.**
- It protects the internal **tissue** against microorganism invasions, abrasions, and UV radiation.

Play audio to learn more.

A third-degree burn will burn the skin down to the bone. Predict three complications.

How does albinism relate to pigmentation?

SMALL INTESTINE

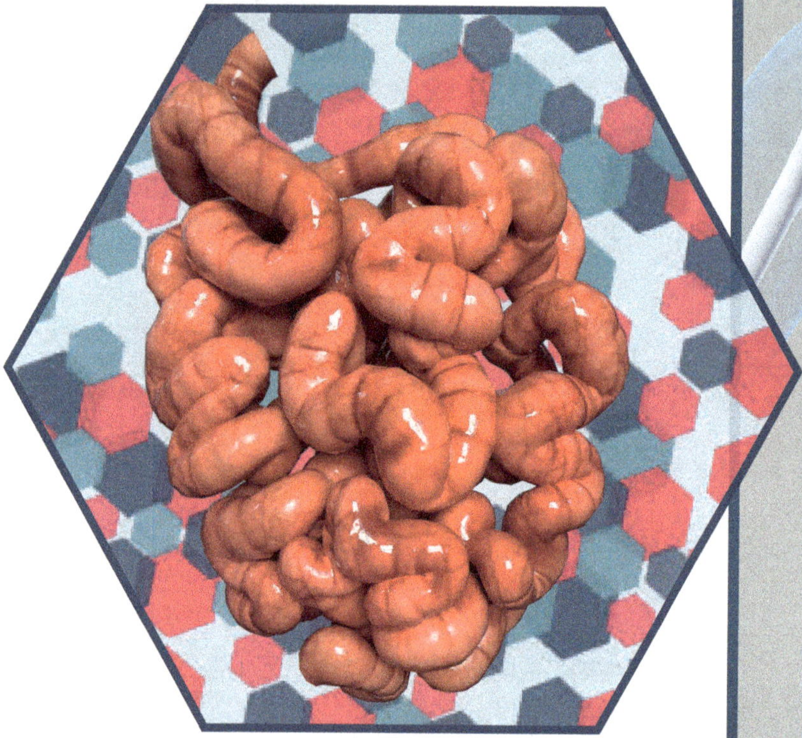

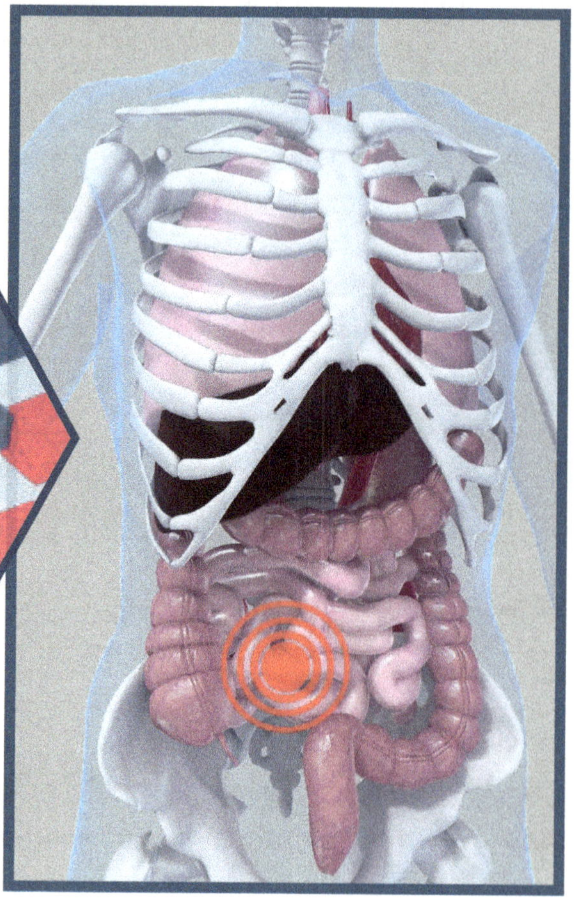

Key Features

- The small intestine is a vital **organ** of the **digestive system.**
- It secretes and receives enzymes that complete all chemical digestion.
- All nutrient absorption occurs in this **organ.**
- It is the longest portion of the **digestive system,** averaging six to seven meters, with three regions: **duodenum, jejunum,** and **ileum.**

Play audio to learn more.

Functionally why is it important that the small intestine is so long?

Name three organs that secrete into the small intestine.

LARGE INTESTINE

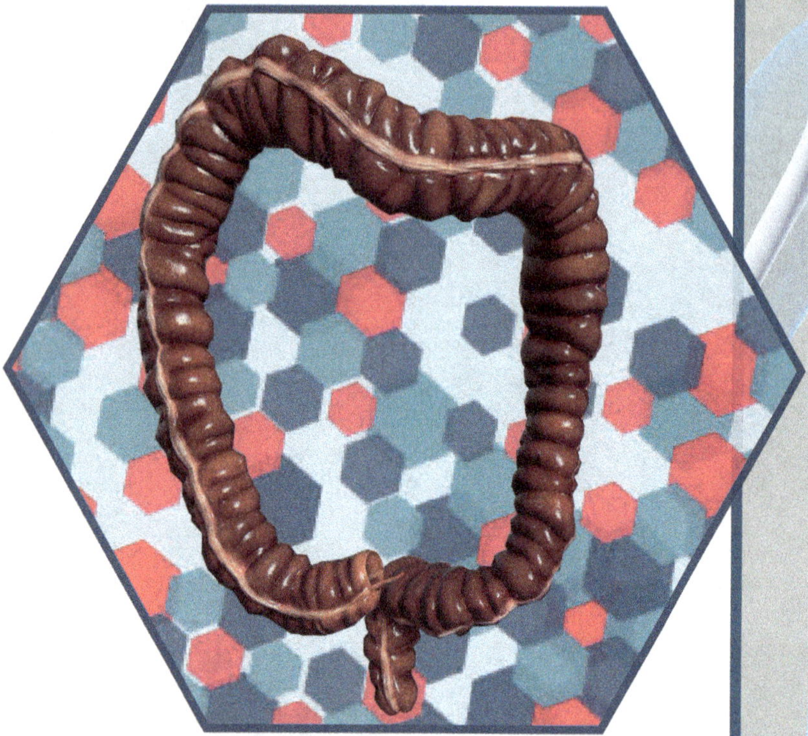

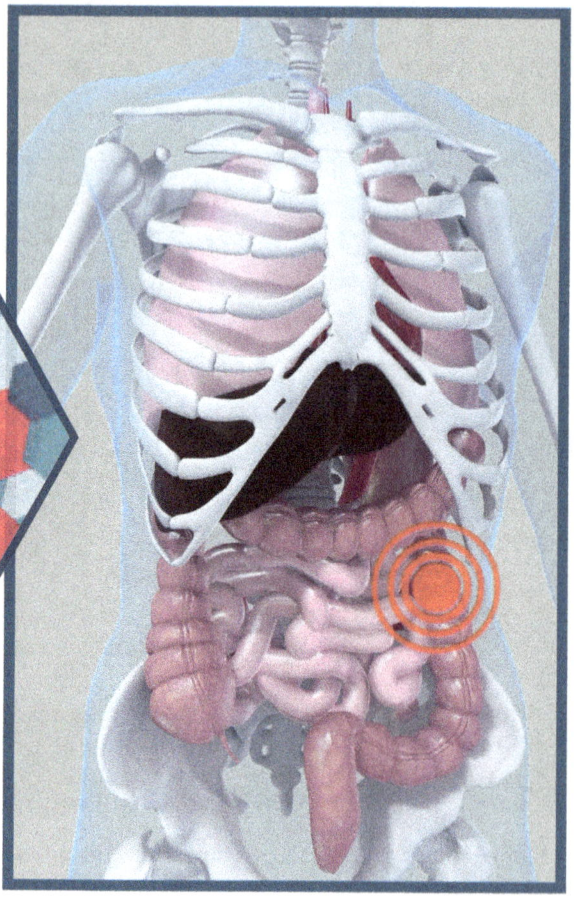

Key Features

- The large intestine is a vital **organ** of the **digestive system.**
- This **organ** is often referred to as the colon.
- It is the site of water and electrolyte reabsorption and feces compaction.
- Averaging one-and-a-half meters in length, it is divided into five regions: ascending, transverse, descending, sigmoid, and rectum.

Play audio to learn more.

Questions & Activities

Explain the benefit of your large intestine's bacterial population.

Sketch a **polyp** on the wall of the intestinal tract. Name the common procedure (for ages 50+) that detects them.

BRAIN

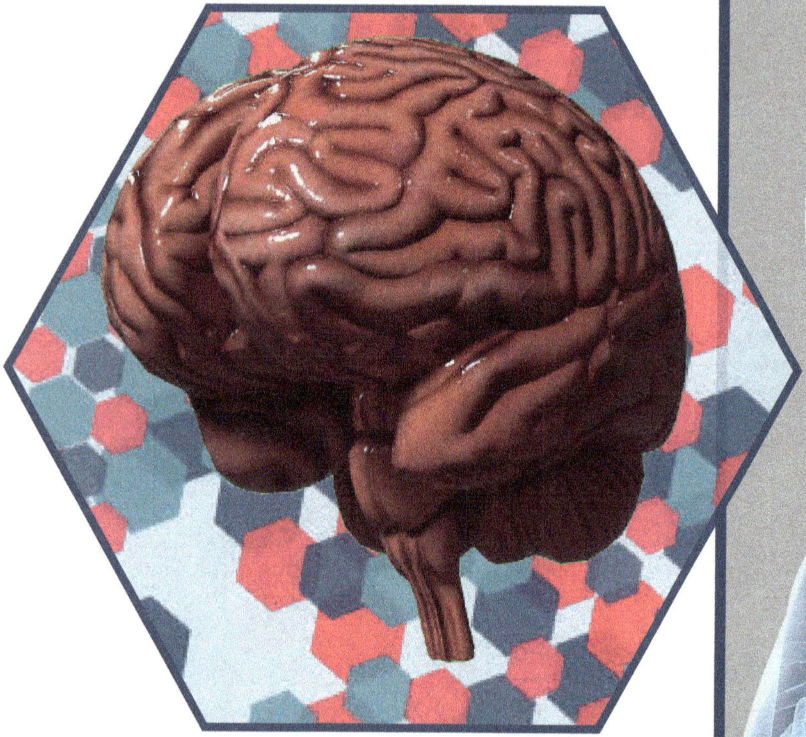

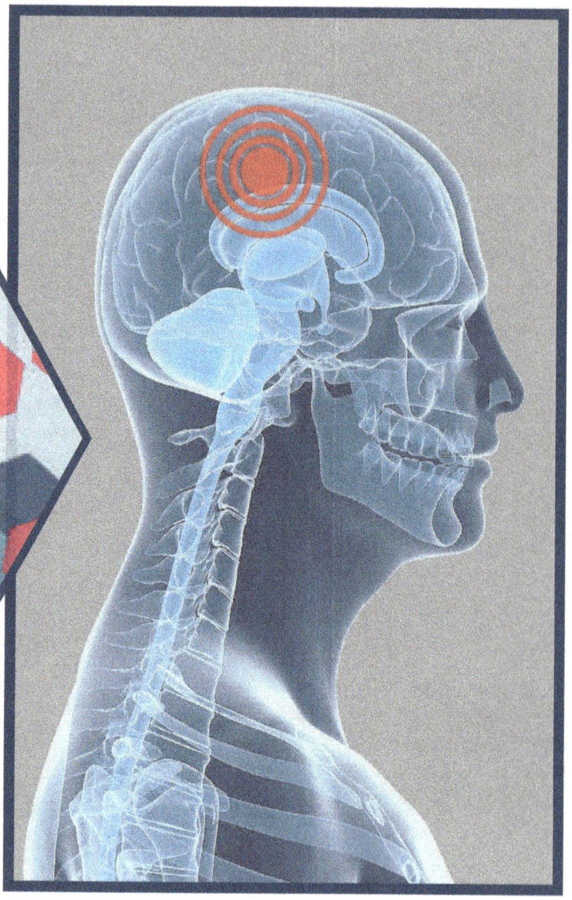

Key Features

- The brain is a vital **organ** of the **nervous system.**
- The main function is to interpret and process information from the five senses.
- It is the control center for all voluntary and involuntary functions of the body.
- This **organ** is divided into three regions: **cerebrum, cerebellum,** and **brainstem.**

Play audio to learn more.

Sketch a brain and label the major lobes of the **cerebrum.**

If a person has a stroke on the right side of the brain, predict two specific symptoms that may occur.

SPLEEN

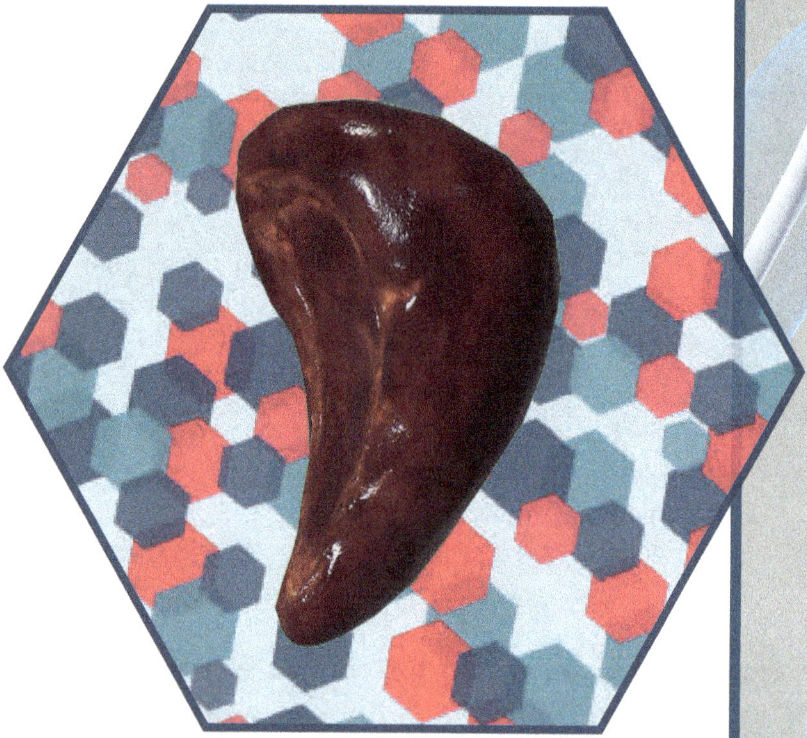

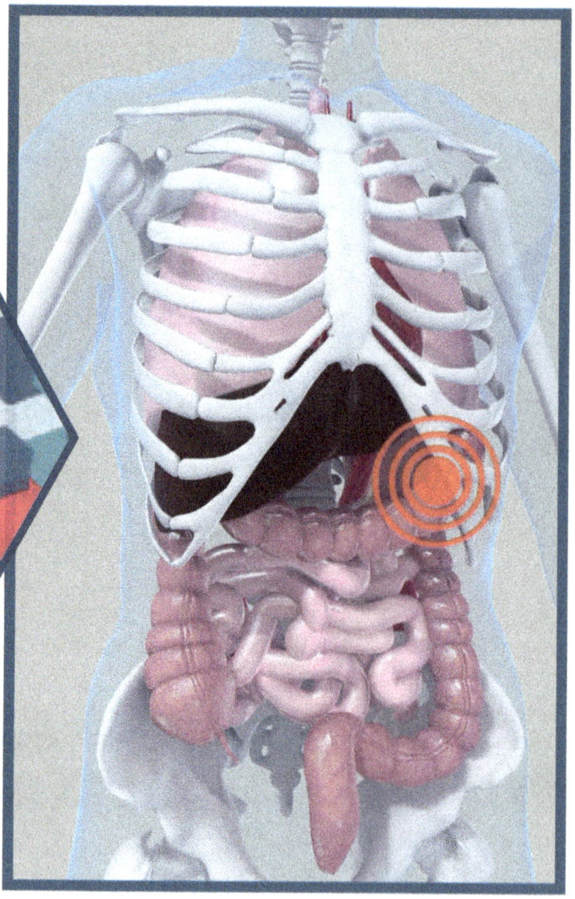

Key Features

- The spleen is a vital **organ** of the **lymphatic system.**
- It filters and recycles old or defective red blood cells.
- This **organ** serves as storage for platelets and white blood cells.
- It is the largest lymphatic **organ** in the body.

Play audio to learn more.

Name two systems the spleen could be considered a part of and why.

What is a splenectomy?

PANCREAS

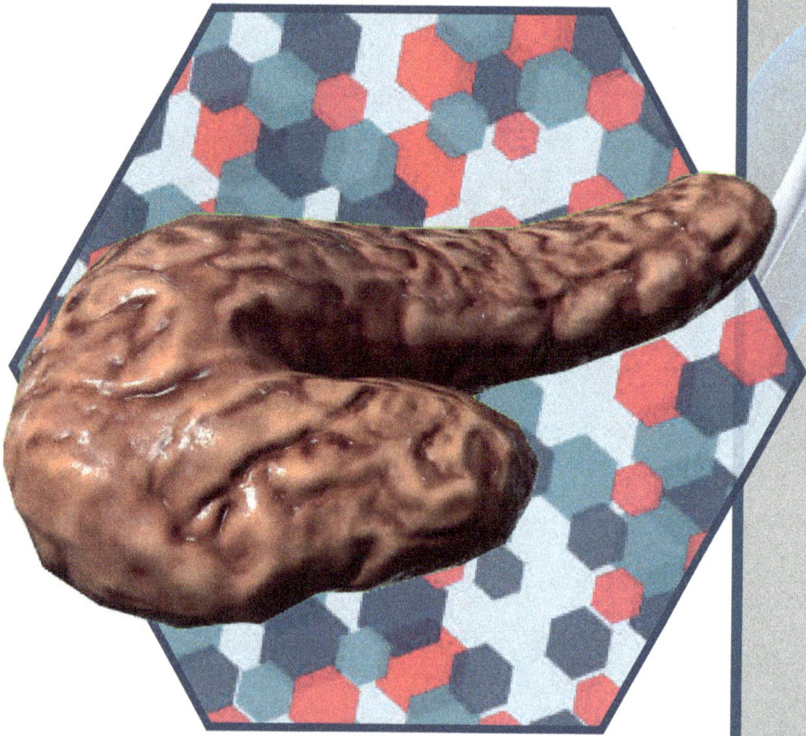

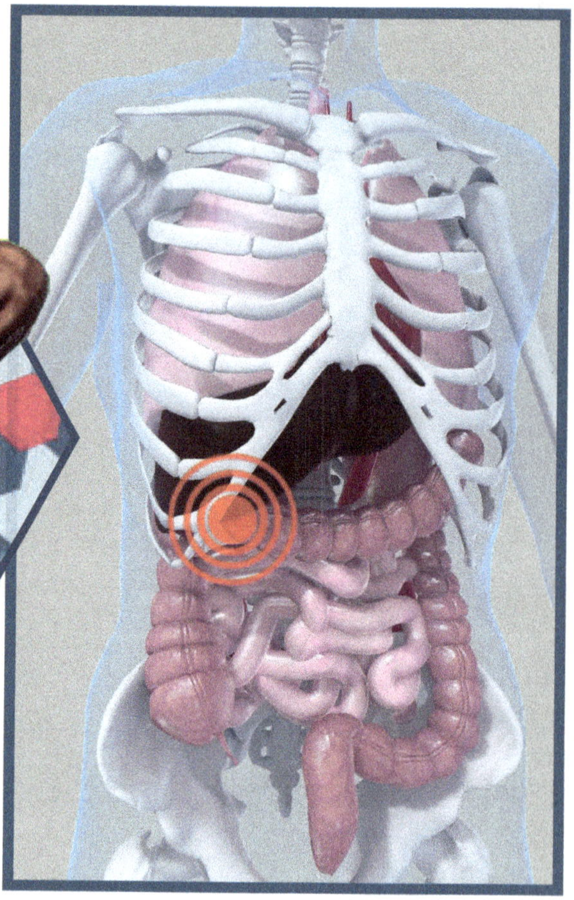

Key Features

- The pancreas is a vital **organ** of both the **lymphatic** and **endocrine systems.**
- It produces and secretes various digestive enzymes.
- This **organ** also produces and secretes the two **hormones insulin** and glucagon.
- It is often referred to as a mixed gland because of its dual roles.

Play audio to learn more.

Is the pancreas more important as an **endocrine** or **exocrine** gland? Why?

Cystic fibrosis can cause mucus to build up around the pancreas. Predict two symptoms.

LIVER

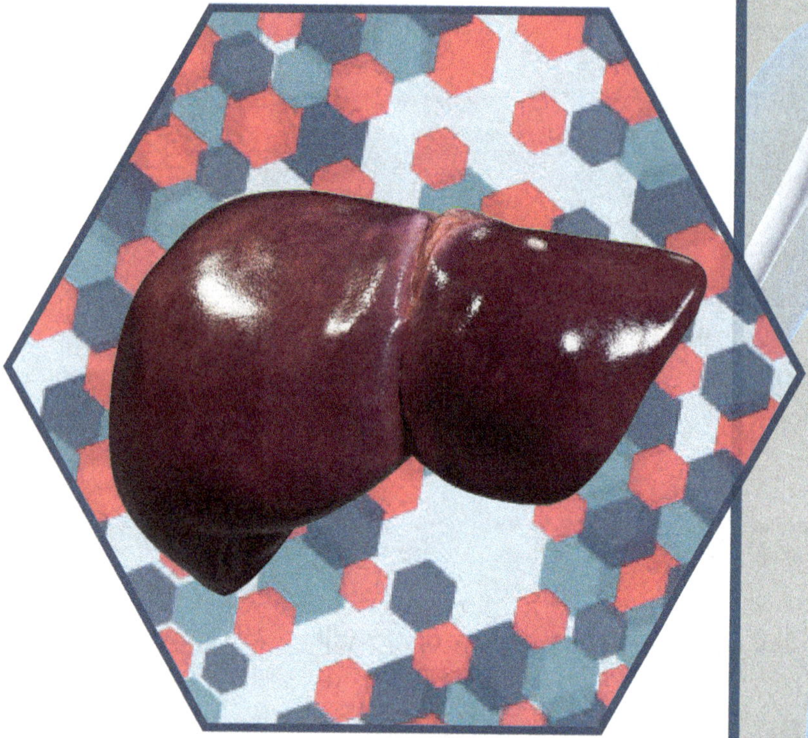

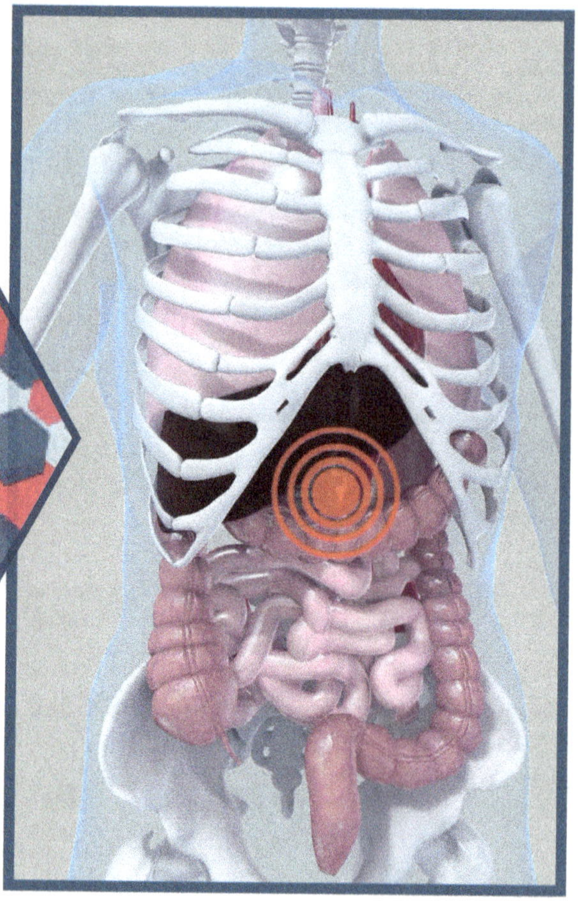

Key Features

- The liver is a vital **organ** of the **digestive system.**
- It is believed to have hundreds of metabolic functions.
- Amongst its functions are detoxifying chemicals in the blood, producing **bile,** and storing **glycogen,** iron, and other vitamins.
- This is the largest gland of the body.

Play audio to learn more.

Questions & Activities

Name three systems the liver could be associated with and what the relationships are.

Could a human survive without a liver? Explain.

GALLBLADDER

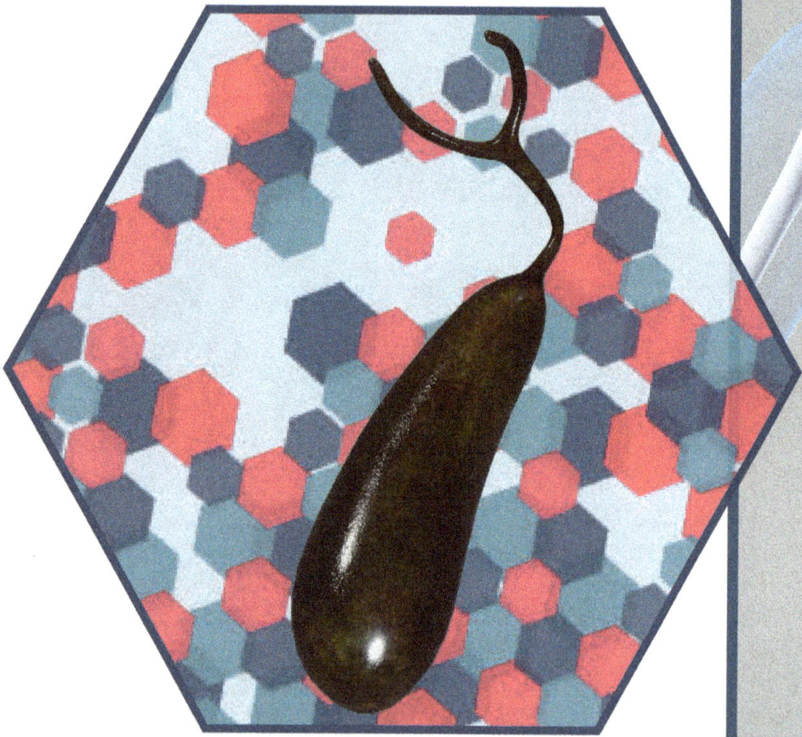

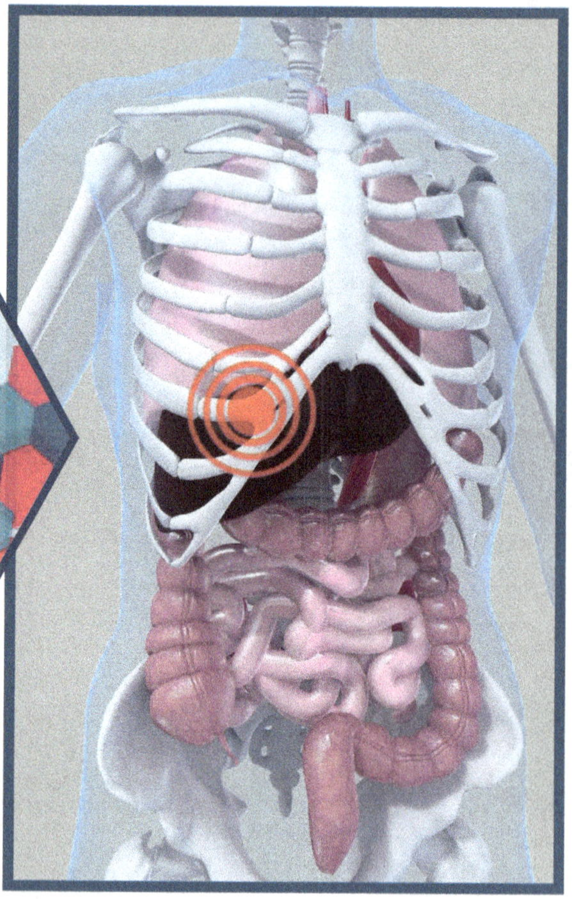

Key Features

- The gallbladder is a vital **organ** of the **digestive system.**
- It stores and concentrates **bile** that the liver produces.
- This **organ** squeezes **bile** into the small intestine when triggered.
- It is located on the underside of the liver but has its own **duct.**

Play audio to learn more.

With what specific type of food digestion would a **gallstone** interfere? Why?

Why is the structure of the gallbladder significant to its function?

EAR

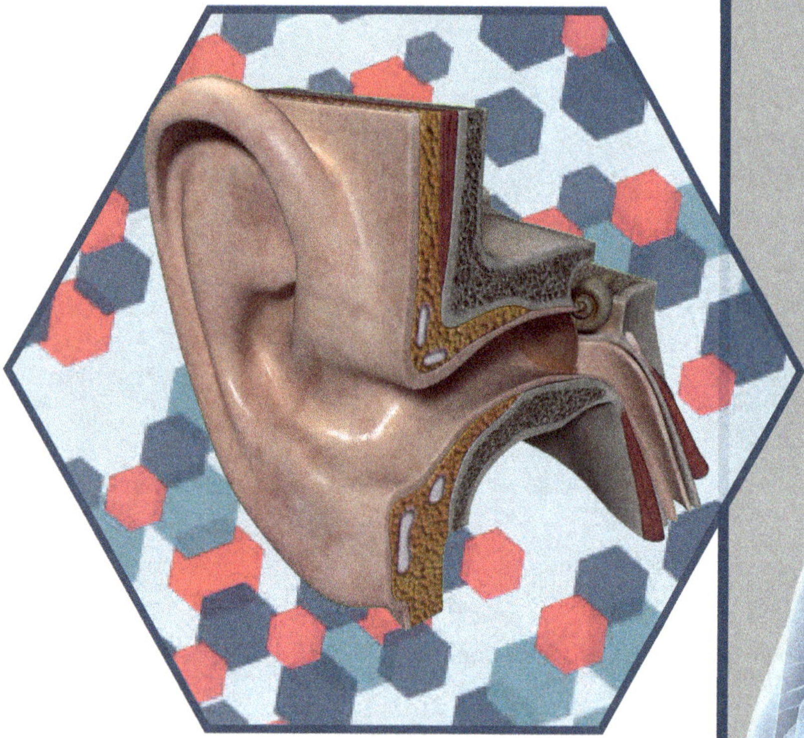

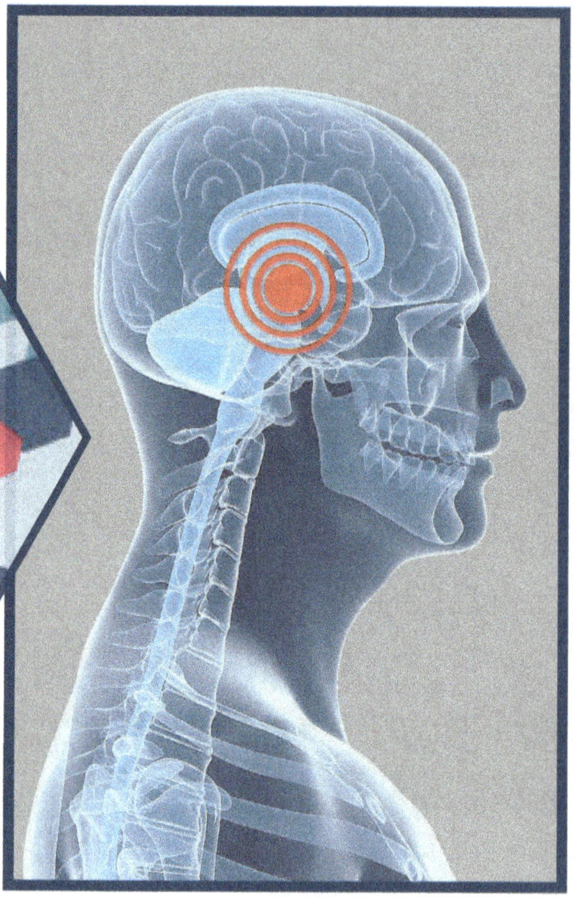

Key Features

- The ear is a vital **organ** of the **nervous system.**
- This **organ** is responsible for hearing and balance.
- It is divided into three regions: external, middle, and inner.
- The three smallest bones in the body are located here.

Play audio to learn more.

Questions & Activities

Sketch the three regions of the ear. Draw arrows indicating the flow of sound waves throughout the ear.

Label all structures with which the sound waves would interact.

EYE

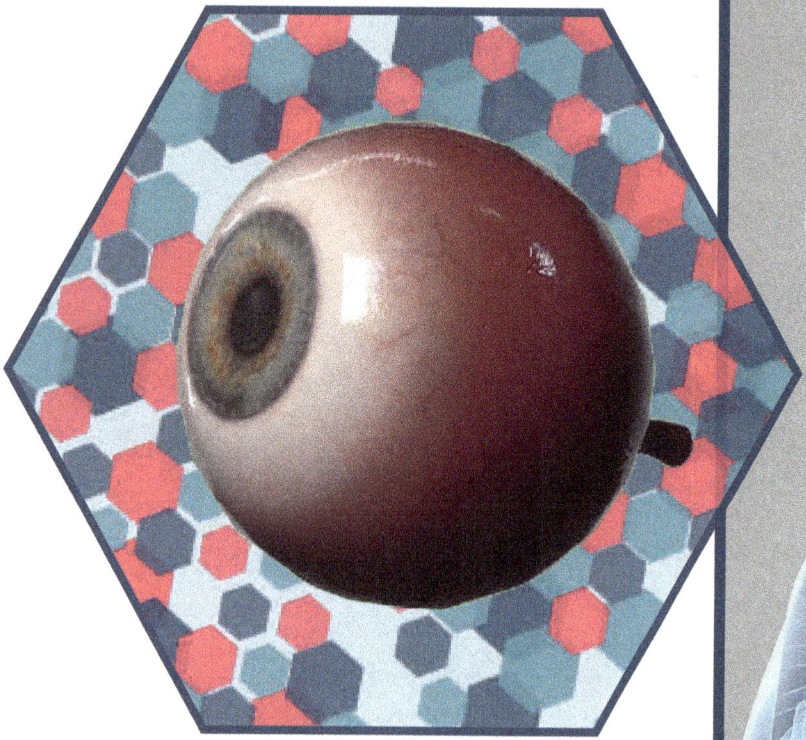

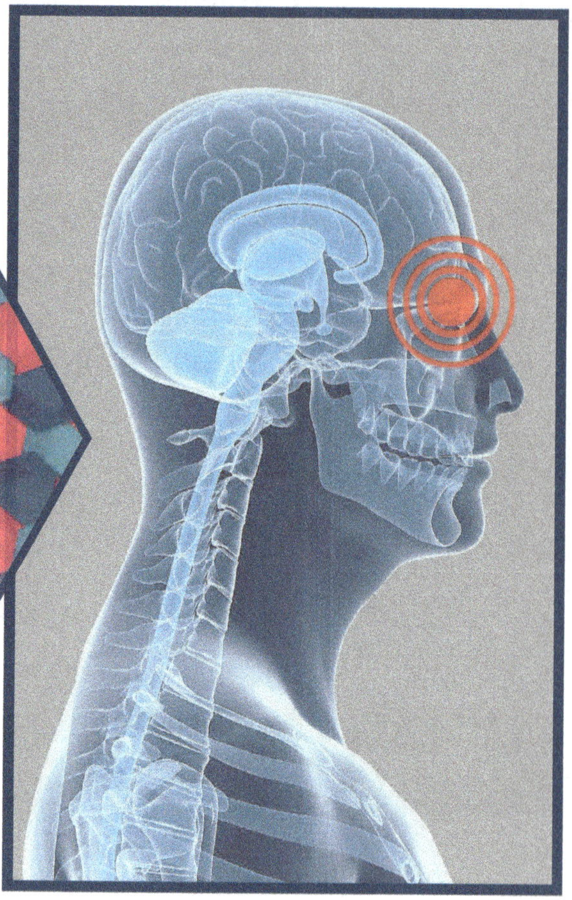

Key Features

- The eye is a vital **organ** of the **nervous system.**
- This **organ** is responsible for sight.
- It contains photoreceptor cells, rods, and cones for both color vision and night vision.
- About 70% of all human sensory receptors are found in the eye.

Play audio to learn more.

The eye is often compared to a camera. Explain this analogy.

What is a cataract? How is it treated?

THYROID

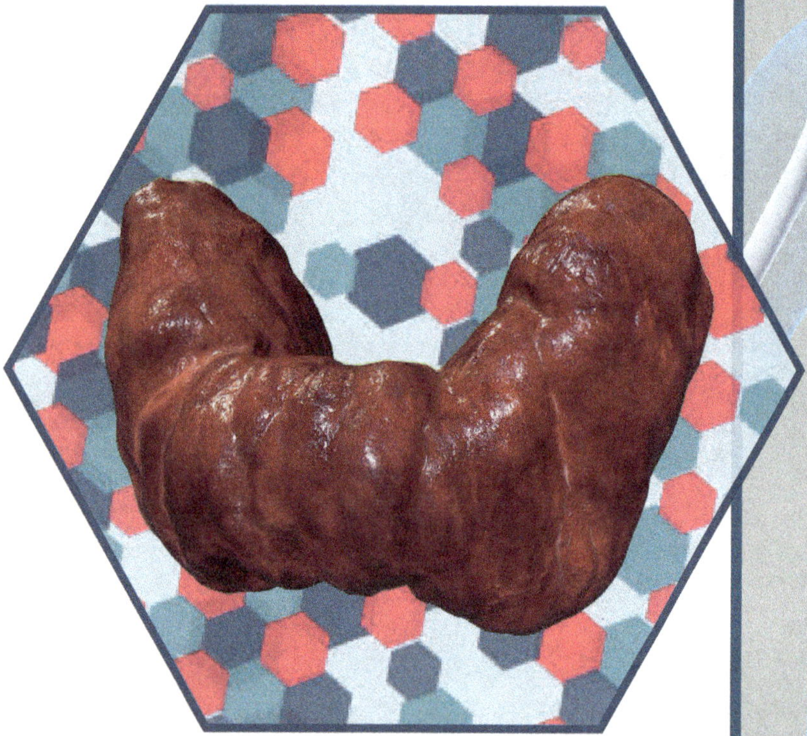

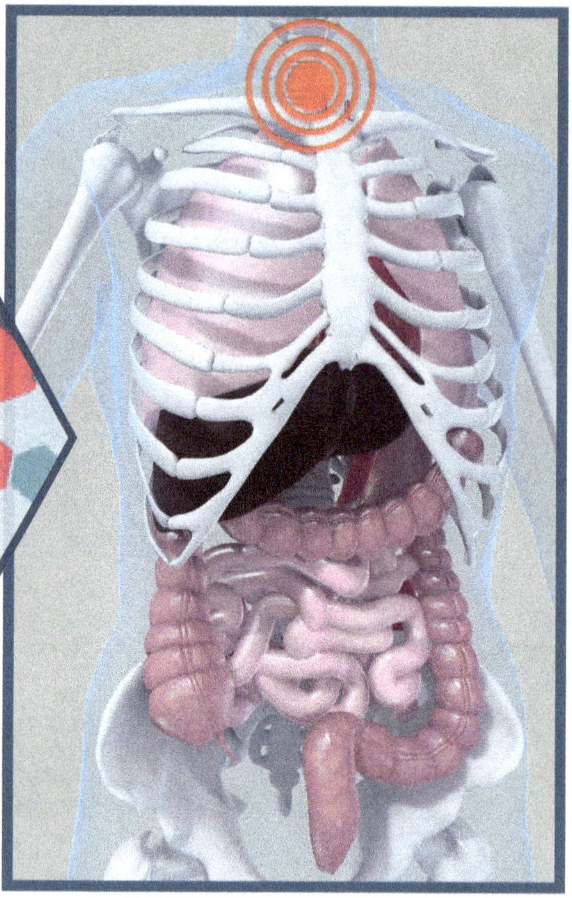

Key Features

- The thyroid is a vital **organ** of the **endocrine system.**
- Its **hormones** regulate the body's **metabolism.**
- This **organ** requires iodine to produce **hormones.**
- It is a unique butterfly-shaped gland on the trachea.

Play audio to learn more.

Can you live without your thyroid? Explain.

What is the connection between iodine and the thyroid's **hormones**?

THYMUS

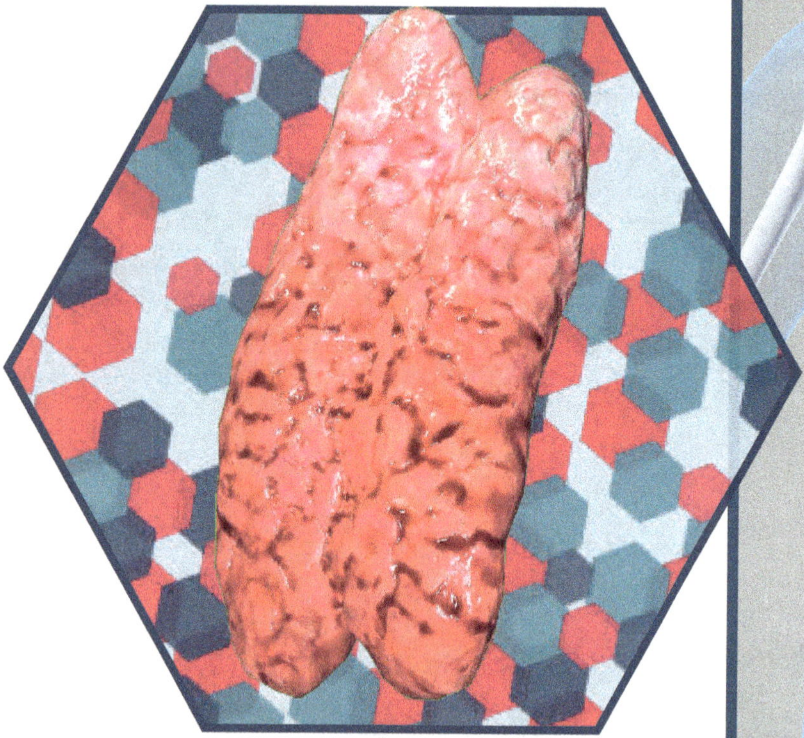

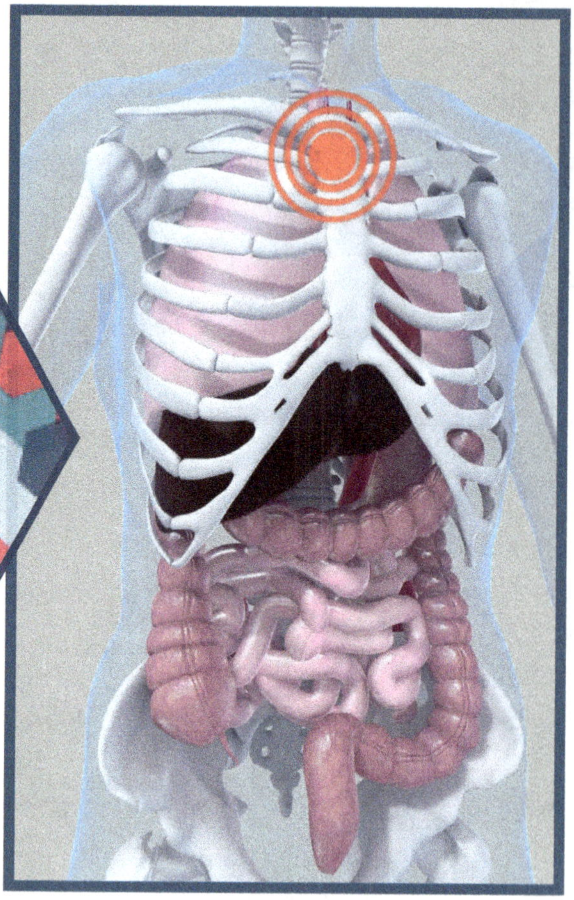

Key Features

- The thymus is a vital **organ** of both the **endocrine** and **immune systems.**
- It is large early in life and atrophies as a person ages.
- This **organ** secretes thymosin (a protein).
- Thymosin helps T-cells become functional in the body.

Play audio to learn more.

Removal of a newborn's thymus would be life-threatening. Why?

What two systems is the thymus considered a part of and how is it associated with each one?

ADRENAL GLANDS

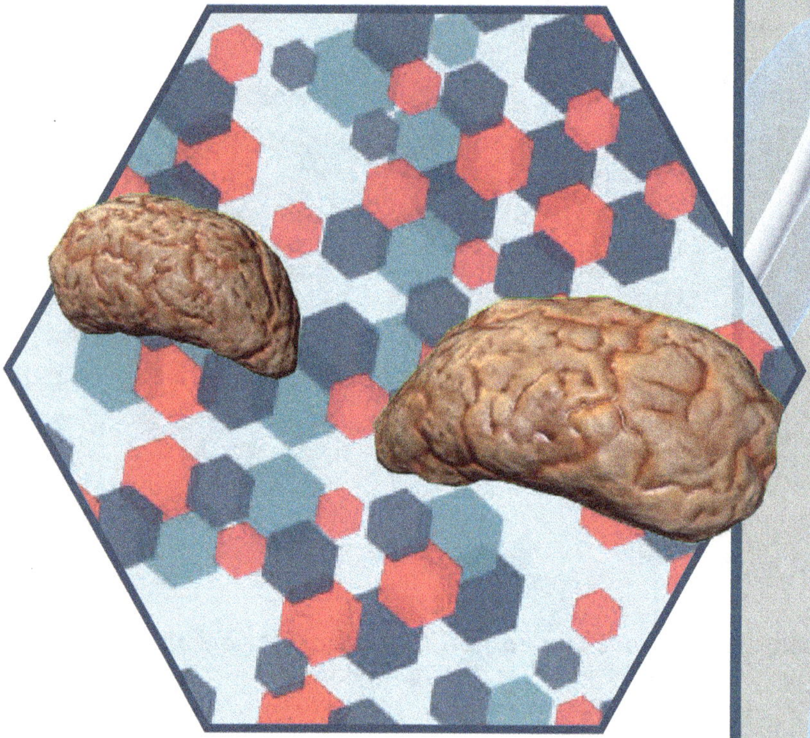

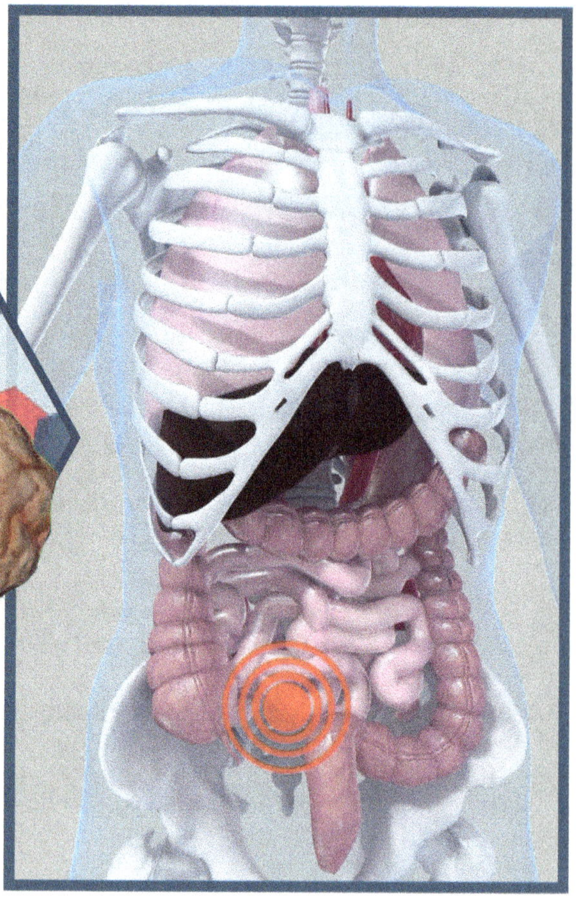

Key Features

- The adrenal glands are a vital **organ** of the **endocrine system.**
- It has two regions: adrenal cortex and adrenal medulla.
- The adrenal cortex secretes **cortisol** and **aldosterone** to help with sugar and mineral **homeostasis.**
- The medulla secretes **epinephrine** (**adrenaline**) which triggers the fight-or-flight response.

Play audio to learn more.

The adrenal glands secrete **adrenaline** to regulate the fight or flight response. Give one personal example of this.

Starvation would trigger which region of the adrenal glands? Why?

TESTES

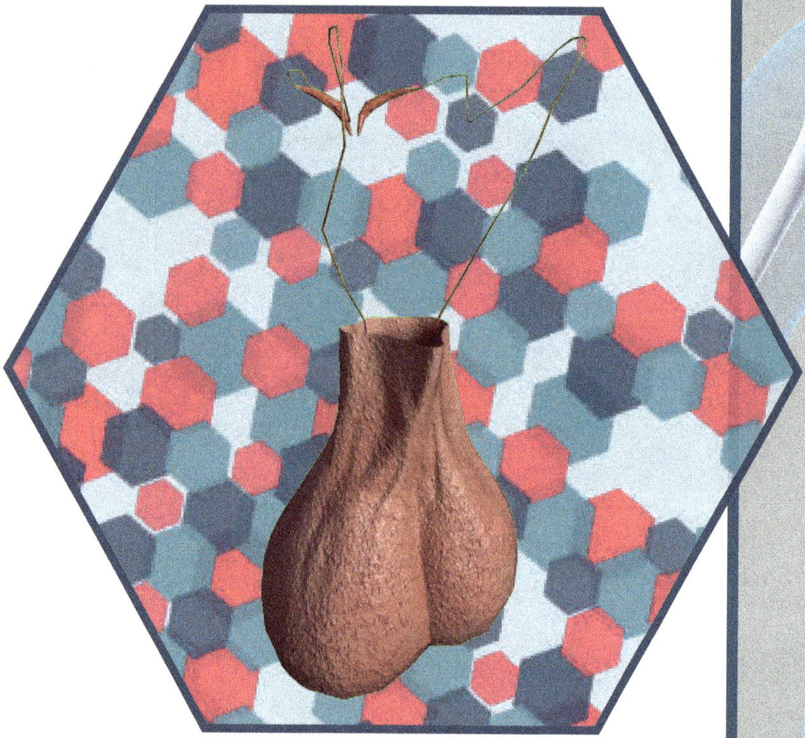

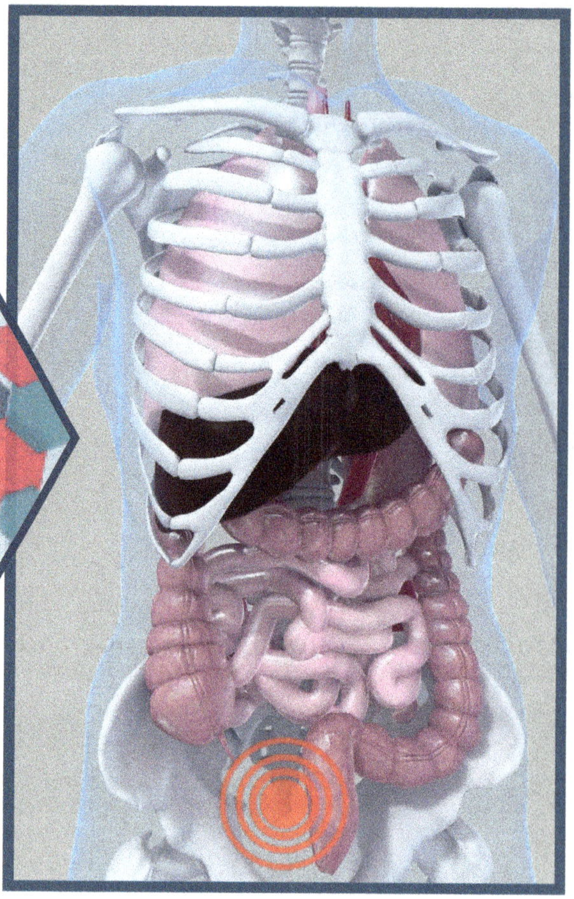

Key Features

- The testes is a vital **organ** of both the **reproductive** and **endocrine systems.**
- Its reproductive function is the production of sperm cells.
- Its **endocrine** function is the production of **testosterone hormones.**
- This **organ** is located outside of the body, as cooler temperatures aid in sperm production.

Play audio to learn more.

Would the removal of one testicle leave a male sterile? Explain.

Why is it necessary that the testes are located outside of the body?

OVARIES

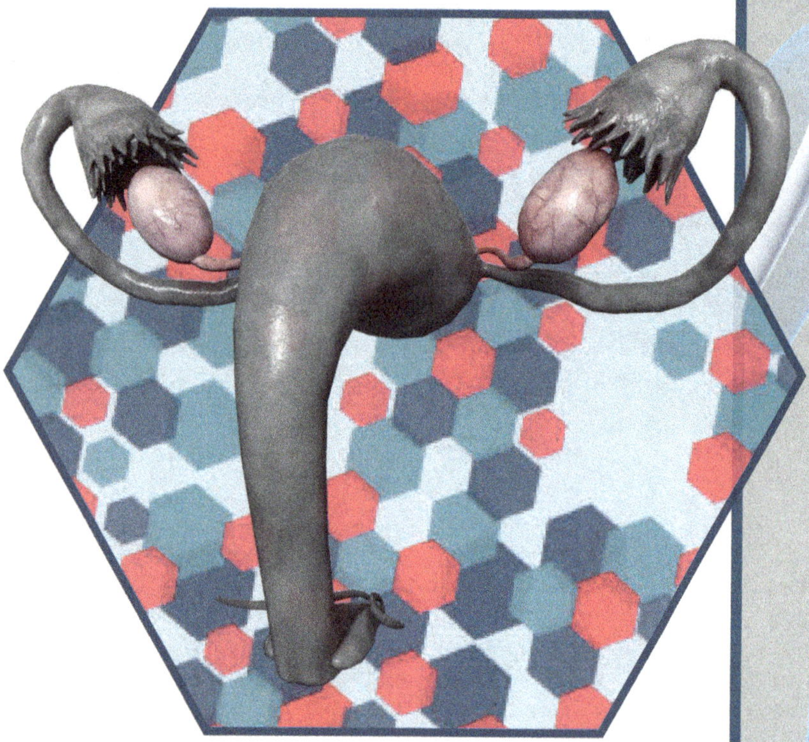

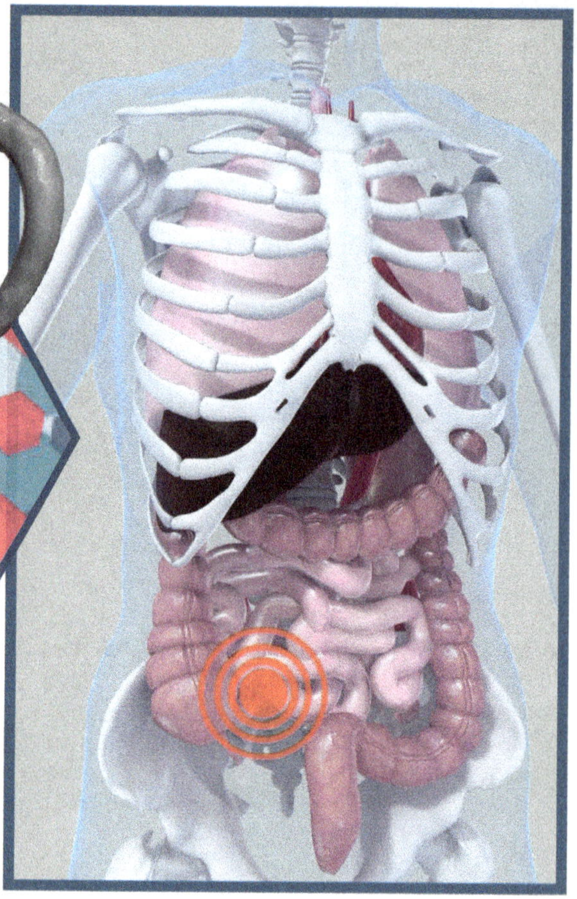

Key Features

- The ovaries are a vital **organ** of both the **reproductive** and **endocrine systems.**
- Its reproductive function is the production of egg cells.
- Its **endocrine** function is the production of **estrogen** and progesterones.
- Starting at puberty, the ovaries release a mature egg through ovulation.

Play audio to learn more.

How do the ovaries facilitate changes in the female body?

The ovaries are homologous to which male structure?

UTERUS

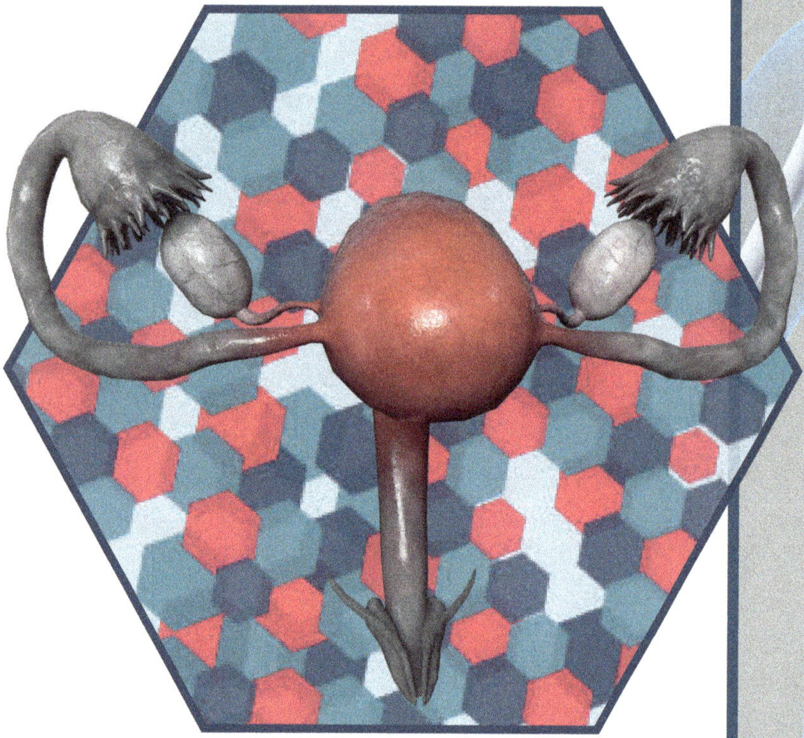

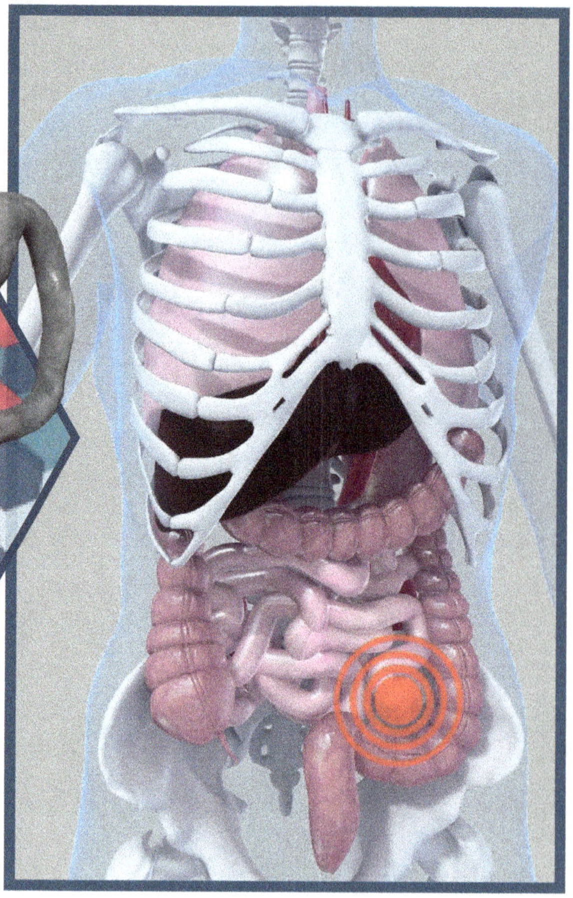

Key Features

- The uterus is a vital **organ** of the **reproductive system.**
- Uterine tubes receive an ovulated egg and move it towards the uterus.
- The uterus receives a fertilized egg and nourishes its embryonic development.
- The uterus is approximately the size and shape of a pear.

Play audio to learn more.

If one of the uterine tubes was blocked, what problems could this cause for a potential pregnancy?

The body of the uterus is expandable. How is this structure related to its potential function?

PITUITARY GLAND

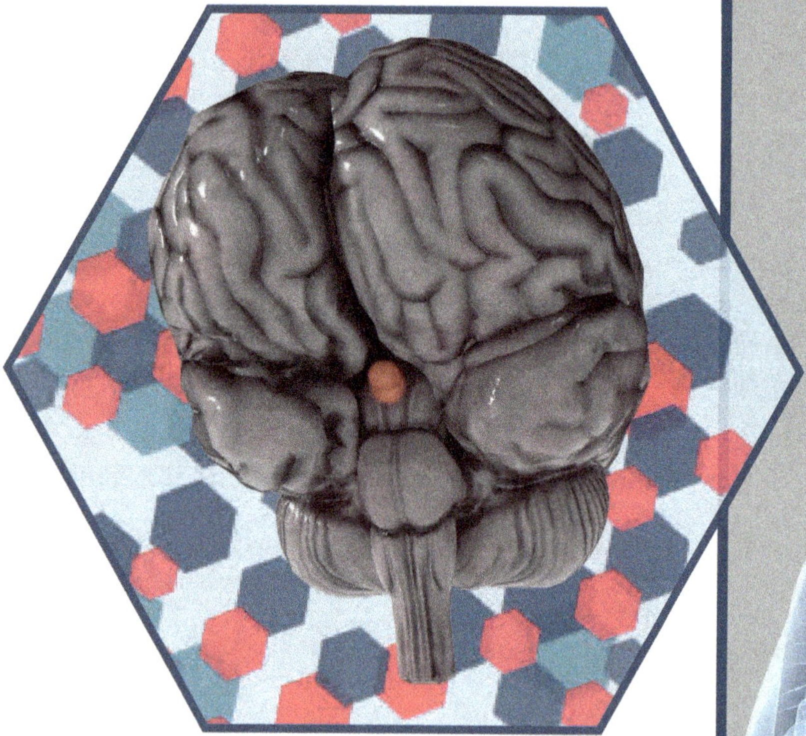

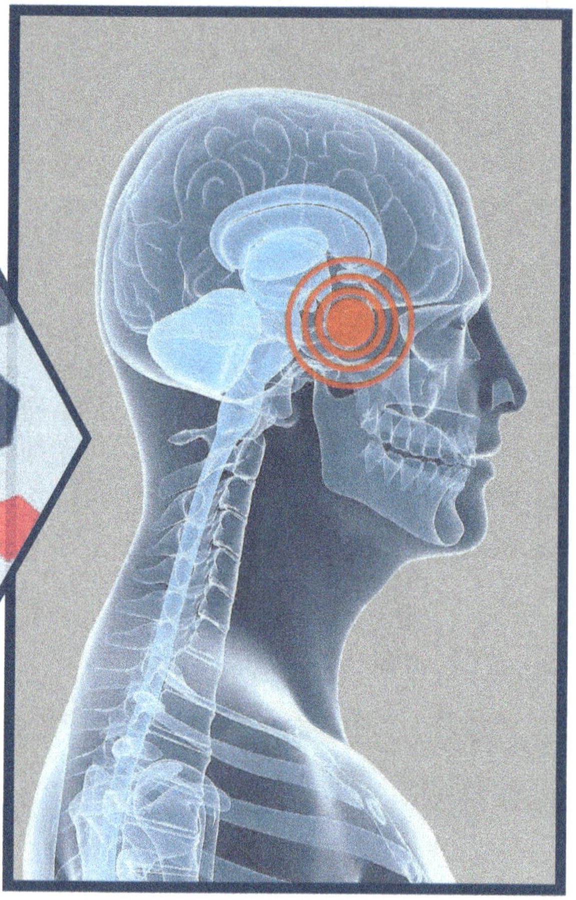

Key Features

- The pituitary gland is a vital **organ** of the **endocrine system.**
- It is often referred to as the "master gland".
- This **organ** secretes many **hormones** that regulate other **endocrine** glands.
- It is divided into two distinct anterior and posterior regions, each with separate functions.

Play audio to learn more.

What causes pituitary dwarfism?

Explain why the pituitary gland is called the "master gland".

SPINAL CORD

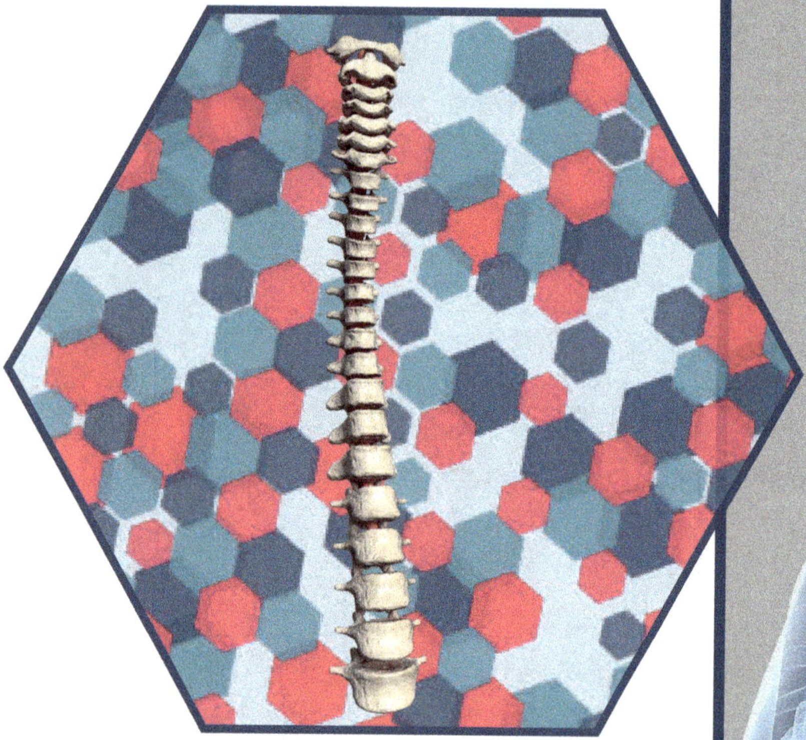

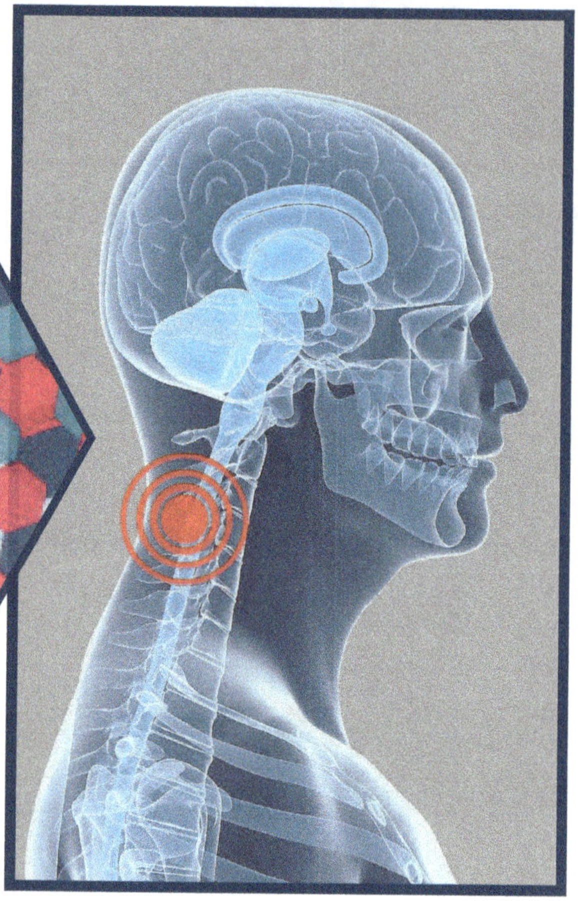

Key Features

- The spinal cord is a vital **organ** of the **nervous system.**
- It serves as a two-way communication between brain and body.
- This **organ** is also a major reflex response center.
- Its composition is similar to an elastic cord; it averages 17 inches in length.

Play audio to learn more.

Questions & Activities

How does the location of an injury along the vertebra determine the degree of possible paralysis?

Sketch a spinal cord and the points in which the spinal nerves originate.

TEETH

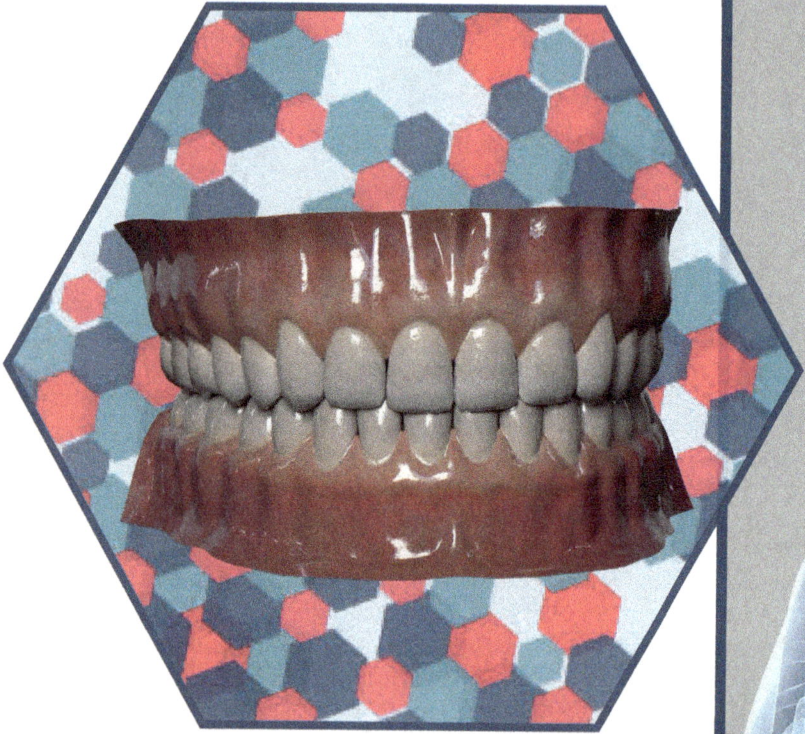

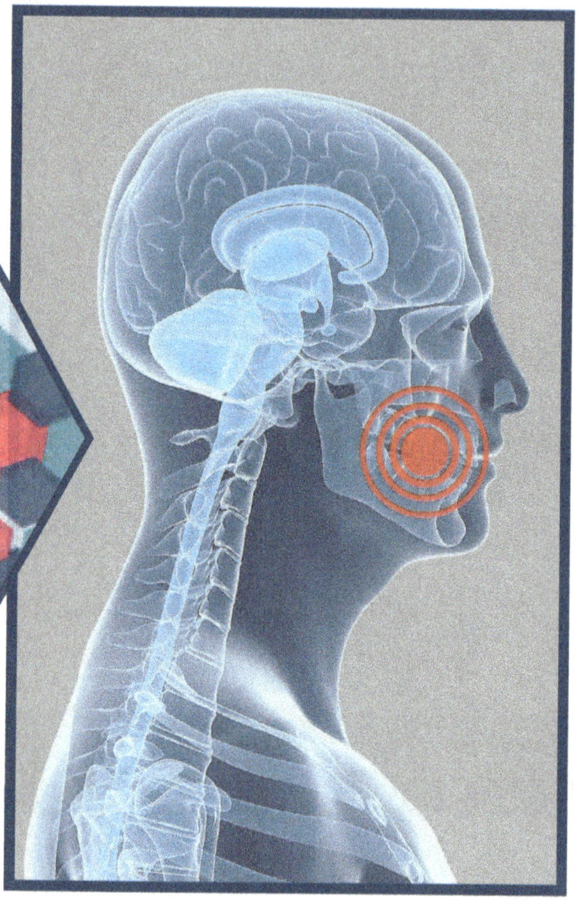

Key Features

- The teeth are a vital **organ** of the **digestive system.**
- There are four types: **incisors, canines, premolars,** and **molars.**
- Their function is to mechanically tear and grind up food.
- Adults have 32 teeth total, if all **wisdom teeth** are present.

Play audio to learn more.

The number of adult teeth can vary from 28 - 32. Why is there a range?

Do humans have homodont or heterodont dentition? Explain.

TONGUE

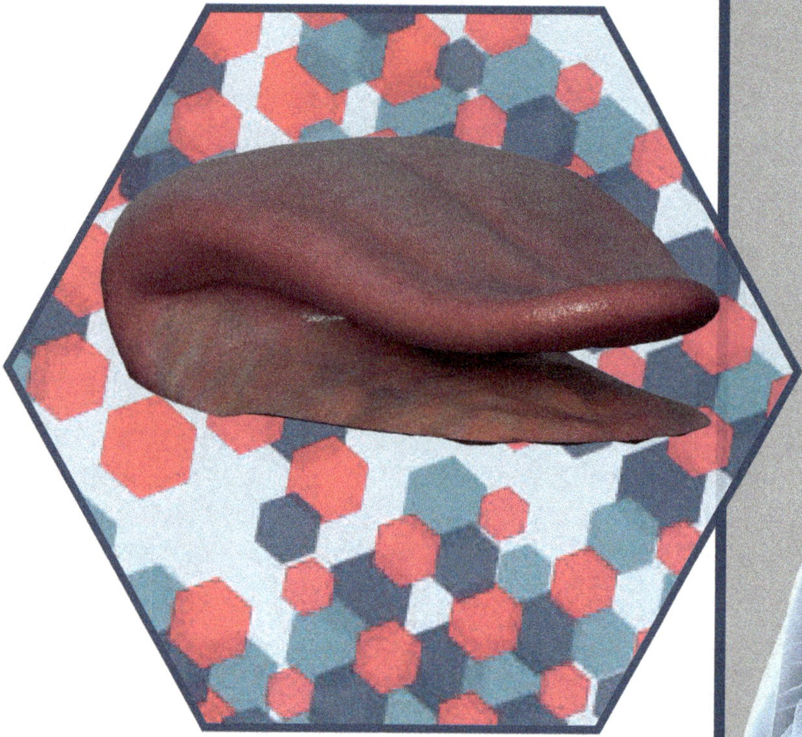

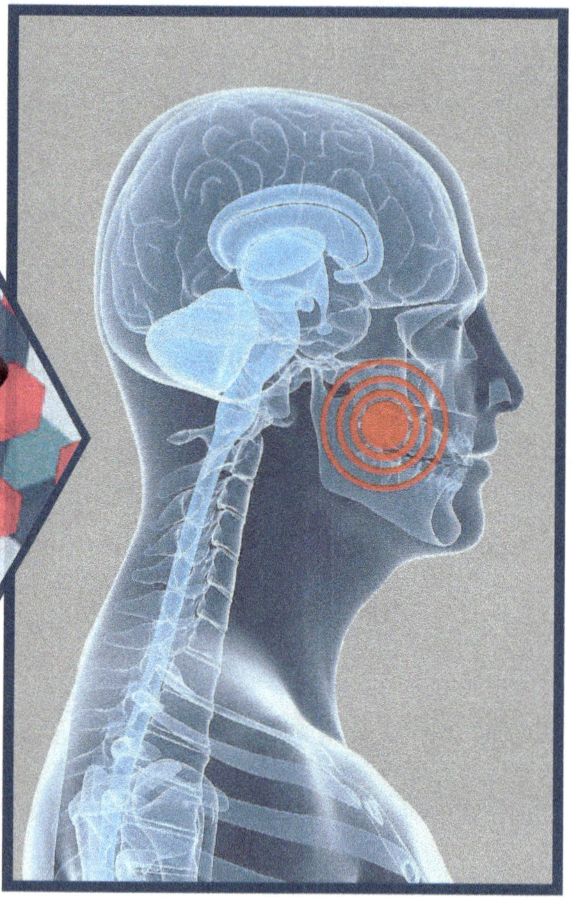

Key Features

- The tongue is a vital **organ** of the **digestive system.**
- This **organ** is involved in chewing, swallowing, tasting, and speaking.
- The top of the tongue is covered in small bumps called **papillae.**
- **Papillae** contain five taste buds: sweet, sour, salty, bitter, and **umami.**

Play audio to learn more.

Sketch the tongue and the location of the five major taste buds. Add labels.

The tongue is involved in speech. Describe how it assists.

LARYNX

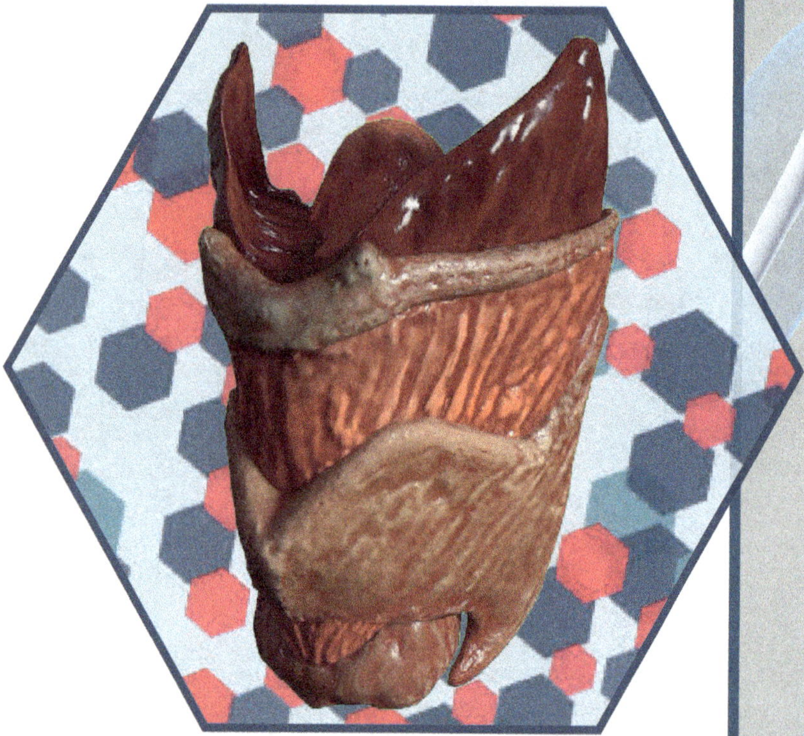

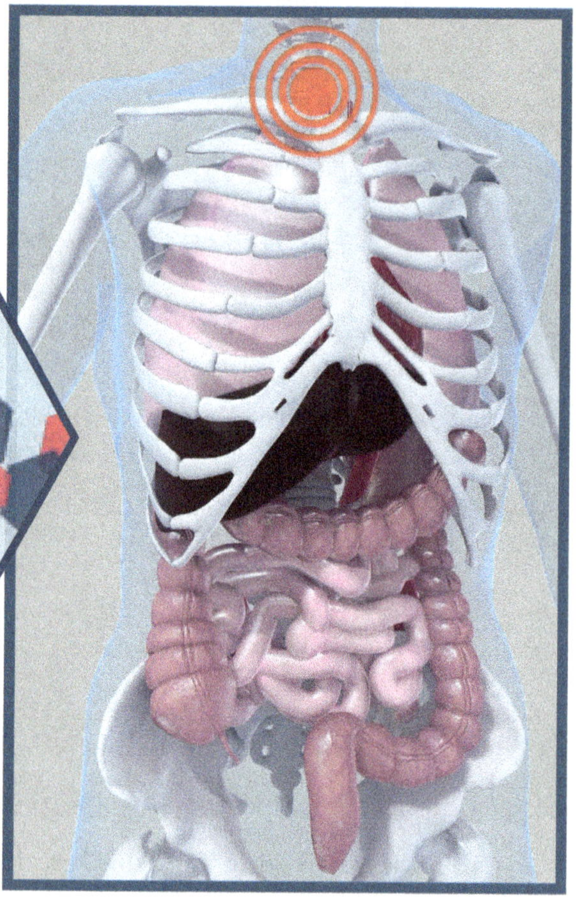

Key Features

- The larynx is a vital **organ** of the **respiratory system.**
- It is blocked by the **epiglottis** during swallowing.
- This **organ** is often referred to as the "voicebox".
- It is vital in producing sounds and speech because it houses the **vocal cords.**

Play audio to learn more.

Why don't females have an Adam's Apple?

List three potential causes of laryngitis.

GLOSSARY

- **adipose** *[ad-uh-pohs]* consisting of, resembling, or relating to fat
- **adrenaline** *[uh-dren-l-in]* a hormone secreted by the adrenal medulla in response to stress
- **aldosterone** *[al-doh-sti-rohn]* a hormone produced by the cortex of the adrenal gland, instrumental in the regulation of sodium and potassium reabsorption in the kidney
- **alveolus** *[al-vee-uh-luhs]* any of the many tiny air sacs of the lungs which allow for rapid gaseous exchange
- **aorta** *[ey-awr-tuh]* the main trunk of the arterial system, moving blood from the left ventricle of the heart to all of the body except the lungs
- **atria** *[ay-tree-uh]* the two upper chambers in the heart, which receive blood from the veins and push it into the ventricles
- **bile** *[bahyl]* a bitter, alkaline, yellow or greenish liquid, secreted by the liver, that aids in absorption and digestion, especially of fats
- **bilirubin** *[bil-uh-roo-bin]* a reddish bile pigment resulting from the breakdown of heme in the liver
- **bolus** *[boh-luh s]* a soft, roundish mass or lump, especially of chewed food
- **brainstem** *[breynstem]* the portion of the brain that is continuous with the spinal cord, functioning in the control of reflexes and essential internal mechanisms such as respiration and heartbeat
- **calcitonin** *[kal-si-toh-nin]* a polypeptide hormone that participates in the regulation of calcium levels in vertebrates by inhibiting loss of calcium from bone to the blood
- **canine** *[key-nahyn]* of or relating to the four pointed teeth situated one on each side of each jaw, next to the incisors
- **carotene** *[kar-uh-teen]* any of three yellow or orange fat-soluble pigments found in many plants and transformed to vitamin A in the liver
- **cerebellum** *[ser-uh-bel-uhm]* a large portion of the brain, serving to coordinate voluntary movements, posture, and balance
- **cerebrum** *[suh-ree-bruhm]* the anterior and largest part of the brain, consisting of two hemispheres and serving to control voluntary movements and coordinate mental actions
- **cholesterol** *[kuh-les-tuh-rohl]* a sterol found in all animal tissues, blood, bile, and animal fats

- **chyme** *[kahym]* the pulpy acidic fluid which passes from the stomach to the small intestine, consisting of gastric juices and partially digested food
- **cilia** *[sil-ee-uh]* minute hairlike organelles, identical in structure to flagella, that line the surfaces of certain cells
- **circulatory system** *[sur-kyuh-ley-toree sis-tuhm]* the system of organs and tissues, including the heart, blood, blood vessels, lymph, lymphatic vessels, and lymph glands, involved in circulating blood and lymph through the body
- **cochlea** *[kok-lee-uh]* a spiral-shaped cavity forming a division of the internal ear in humans and in most other mammals
- **cornea** *[kawr-nee-uh]* the transparent anterior part of the external coat of the eye covering the iris and the pupil
- **cortisol** *[kawr-tuh-sawl]* one of several steroid hormones produced by the adrenal cortex
- **deciduous** *[dih-sij-oo-uhs]* the milk teeth of a mammal, which are shed after a time
- **dermis** *[dur-mis]* the dense inner layer of skin beneath the epidermis, composed of connective tissue, blood and lymph vessels, sweat glands, hair follicles, and an elaborate sensory nerve network
- **dialysis** *[dahy-al-uh-sis]* the process of removing excess water, solutes, and toxins from the blood in people whose kidneys can no longer perform these functions naturally
- **digestive system** *[dih-jes-tiv sis-tuhm]* the system by which ingested food is acted upon by physical and chemical means to provide the body with absorbable nutrients and excrete waste products
- **duct** *[duhkt]* a tube, canal, or vessel conveying a body fluid, especially a glandular secretion or excretion
- **electrolytes** *[ih-lek-truh-lahyts]* a substance that produces an electrically conducting solution when dissolved in water
- **enamel** *[ih-nam-uhl]* hard, calcareous substance covering the exposed portion of a tooth
- **endocrine** *[en-duh-krin]* secreting internally into the blood or lymph
- **enzyme** *[en-zahym]* any of various proteins originating from living cells and capable of producing certain chemical changes in organic substances by catalytic action, as in digestion
- **epidermis** *[ep-i-dur-mis]* the outer, nonvascular, nonsensitive layer of the skin, covering the true skin
- **epiglottis** *[ep-i-glot-is]* a thin, valvelike, cartilaginous structure that covers the glottis during swallowing, preventing the entrance of food and drink into the larynx

- **epinephrine** *[ep-uh-nef-rin]* a hormone secreted by the adrenal medulla upon stimulation by the central nervous system in response to stress, and acting to increase heart rate, blood pressure, cardiac output, and carbohydrate metabolism
- **erythropoietin (EPO)** *[ih-rith-roh-poi-i-tn]* a hormone formed especially in the kidney and stimulating red blood cell formation
- **estrogen** *[es-truh-juhn]* female sex hormones produced primarily by the ovarian follicles of female mammals
- **exocrine** *[ek-suh-krin]* of or relating to an exocrine gland or its secretion
- **gallstone** *[gawl-stohn]* an abnormal stonelike mass, usually of cholesterol, formed in the gallbladder or bile passages
- **gamete** *[gam-eet]* a mature sexual reproductive cell, as a sperm or egg, that unites with another cell to form a new organism
- **glottis** *[glot-is]* the opening at the upper part of the larynx, between the vocal cords
- **gluconeogenesis** *[gloo-koh-nee-uh-jen-uh-sis]* the breakdown of protein and fat for conversion to glucose in the liver
- **glycogen** *[glahy-kuh-juhn]* a white, tasteless polysaccharide similar to starch, constituting the principal carbohydrate storage material in animals and occurring chiefly in the liver, muscle, and in fungi and yeasts
- **hemoglobin** *[hee-muh-gloh-bin]* the oxygen-carrying pigment of red blood cells that gives them their red color and serves to convey oxygen to the tissues
- **homeostasis** *[hoh-mee-uh-stey-sis]* the state of steady internal physical and chemical conditions maintained by living systems
- **hormone** *[hawr-mohn]* any of various internally secreted compounds formed in endocrine glands, that affect the functions of specifically receptive organs or tissues when transported to them by the body fluids
- **hypothalamus** *[hahy-puh-thal-uh-muhs]* a region of the brain that functions as the main control center for the autonomic nervous system by regulating sleep cycles, body temperature, appetite, etc., and that acts as an endocrine gland by producing hormones
- **immunocompetent** *[im-yuh-noh-kom-pi-tnt]* capable of developing immunity after exposure to antigens
- **incisor** *[in-sahy-zer]* any of the four anterior teeth in each jaw, used for cutting and gnawing
- **incus** *[ing-kuhs]* the middle one of a chain of three small bones in the middle ear of humans and other mammals
- **insulin** *[in-suh-lin]* a hormone produced in the pancreas that regulates the metabolism of glucose and other nutrients

- **integumentary system** *[in-teg-yuh-men-tuh-ree sis-tuhm]* comprises the skin and its appendages acting to protect the body from various kinds of damage, such as loss of water or injury from the outside
- **iris** *[ahy-ris]* the colored portion of the eye that contains a circular opening, the pupil, in its center
- **ligament** *[lig-uh-muhnt]* a band of tissue, usually white and fibrous, serving to connect bones, and hold organs in place
- **lymphatic system** *[lim-fat-ik sis-tuhm]* composed of a large network of lymphatic vessels that carry a clear fluid called lymph directionally towards the heart
- **malleus** *[mal-ee-uhs]* the outermost of a chain of three small bones in the middle ear of mammals
- **marrow** *[mar-oh]* a soft, fatty, vascular tissue in the interior cavities of bones that is a major site of blood cell production
- **melanin** *[mel-uh-nin]* an insoluble pigment, found in all forms of animal life, that accounts for the dark color of skin, hair, fur, scales, feathers, etc.
- **menstruation** *[men-stroo-ey-shuhn]* the periodic discharge of blood and mucosal tissue from the uterus, occurring approximately monthly from puberty to menopause in nonpregnant women and females of other primate species
- **metabolism** *[muh-tab-uh-liz-uhm]* physical and chemical processes in an **organ**ism by which its material substance is produced, maintained, and destroyed, and by which energy is made available
- **molar** *[moh-ler]* a tooth having a broad biting surface adapted for grinding, being one of twelve in humans, with three on each side of the upper and lower jaws
- **muscular system** *[muhs-kyuh-ler sis-tuhm]* an organ system consisting of skeletal, smooth, and cardiac muscles that permits movement of the body, maintains posture, and circulates blood throughout the body
- **nephron** *[nef-ron]* a functional unit of the kidney that filters blood, reabsorbs substances, and excretes nitrogenous waste and excess water and salts in the form of urine
- **nervous system** *[nur-vuhs sis-tuhm]* a complex collection of nerves and specialized cells known as neurons that transmit signals between different parts of the body
- **organ** *[awr-guhn]* a grouping of tissues into a distinct structure, as a heart or kidney in animals that performs a specialized task
- **ovulate** *[ov-yuh-leyt]* to produce and discharge eggs from the ovary or ovarian follicle
- **papilla** *[puh-pil-uh]* any small, nipplelike process or projection

- **paralysis** *[puh-ral-uh-sis]* a loss or impairment of voluntary movement in a body part, caused by injury or disease of the nerves, brain, or spinal cord
- **pathogen** *[path-uh-juhn]* any disease-producing agent, especially a virus, bacterium, or other microorganism
- **pepsin** *[pep-sin]* an enzyme, produced in the stomach
- **pericardium** *[per-i-kahr-dee-uhm]* the conical sac of serous membrane that encloses the heart and the roots of the great blood vessels of vertebrates
- **peristalsis** *[per-uh-stawl-sis]* the progressive wave of contraction and relaxation of a tubular muscular system, especially the alimentary canal, by which the contents are forced through the system
- **phrenic nerve** *[fren-ik nurv]* a nerve that arises mainly from the fourth cervical nerve and is primarily the motor nerve of the diaphragm but also sends sensory fibers to the pericardium
- **platelet** *[pleyt-lit]* a small platelike body, especially a blood platelet
- **polyp** *[pol-ip]* a projecting growth from a mucous surface being either a tumor or hypertrophy of the mucous membrane
- **premolar** *[pree-moh-ler]* any of eight teeth located in pairs on each side of the upper and lower jaws between the cuspids and molar teeth
- **progesterone** *[proh-jes-tuh-rohn]* a hormone that prepares the uterus for the fertilized ovum and maintains pregnancy
- **pulmonary trunk** *[puhl-muh-ner-ee truhngk]* an arterial trunk with origin from the right ventricle of the heart, and dividing into the right and left pulmonary arteries, which enter the corresponding lungs and branch with the bronchi
- **pupil** *[pyoo-puhl]* the expanding and contracting opening in the iris of the eye, through which light passes to the retina
- **pyloric valve** *[pahy-lawr-ick valv]* a fold of mucous membrane at the gastroduodenal junction, enclosing the pylorus
- **reproductive system** *[ree-pruh-duhk-tiv sis-tuhm]* a system of sex organs within an **organ**ism which work together for the purpose of sexual reproduction
- **respiratory system** *[res-per-uh-tawr-ee sis-tuhm]* a biological system consisting of specific organs and structures used for gas exchange
- **retina** *[ret-n-uh]* the innermost coat of the posterior part of the eyeball that receives the image produced by the lens, is continuous with the optic nerve, and consists of several layers, one of which contains the rods and cones that are sensitive to light
- **rugae** *[roo-jee]* wrinkles, folds, or ridges
- **scrotum** *[skroh-tuhm]* the pouch of skin that contains the testes
- **skeletal system** *[skel-i-tl sis-tuhm]* all of the bones and joints in the body providing support and protection for the soft tissues that make up the rest of the body

- **sphincter** *[sfingk-ter]* a circular band of voluntary or involuntary muscle that encircles an orifice of the body or one of its hollow organs
- **stapes** *[stey-peez]* the innermost, stirrup-shaped bone of a chain of three small bones in the middle ear involved in the conduction of sound vibrations to the inner ear
- **stereocilia** *[ster-ee-uh-sil-ee-uhm]* any of the long, flexible microvilli that superficially resemble cilia and occur as a brush border or series of tufts on the surface of various epithelial tissues
- **sterile** *[ster-il]* free from living germs or microorganisms
- **testosterone** *[tes-tos-tuh-rohn]* the sex hormone secreted by the testes, that stimulates the development of male sex organs, secondary sexual traits, and sperm
- **thoracic cavity** *[thaw-ras-ik kav-i-tee]* the space within the walls of the chest, bounded below by the diaphragm and above by the neck, and containing the heart and lungs
- **tissue** *[tish-oo]* an aggregate of similar cells and cell products forming a definite kind of structural material with a specific function, in a multicellular organism
- **umami** *[oo-mah-mee]* a strong meaty taste imparted by glutamate and certain other amino acids: often considered to be one of the basic taste sensations along with sweet, sour, bitter, and salty
- **urinary system** *[yoo r-uh-ner-ee sis-tuhm]* consists of the kidneys, ureters, bladder, and the urethra to eliminate waste from the body, regulate blood volume and blood pressure, control levels of electrolytes and metabolites, and regulate blood pH
- **vasectomy** *[va-sek-tuh-mee]* excision of the vas deferens, or of a portion of it to affect sterility in men
- **vena cava** *[vee-nuh key-vuh]* either of two large veins discharging blood into the right atrium of the heart, one (superior vena cava or precava) conveying blood from the head, chest, and upper extremities and the other (inferior vena cava or postcava) conveying blood from all parts below the diaphragm
- **ventricles** *[ven-tri-kuhlz]* either of the two lower chambers on each side of the heart that receive blood from the atria and in turn force it into the arteries
- **vessel** *[ves-uhl]* a tube or duct, as an artery or vein, containing or conveying blood or some other body fluid
- **villi** *[vil-iy]* wormlike process on certain membranes, especially on the mucous membrane of the small intestine, where they serve in absorbing nutriment
- **vocal cords** *[voh-kuhl kawrdz]* either of the two pairs of folds of mucous membrane projecting into the cavity of the larynx
- **wisdom teeth** *[wiz-duhm teeth]* the third molar on each side of the upper and lower jaws and the last type of teeth to erupt

NEXT GENERATION SCIENCE STANDARDS

Aligning teaching and learning to the NGSS allows teachers to ensure students' learning occurs in conjunction with the existing science curricula. The content and activities in this augmented reality (AR) lab book have the potential to address any or all of the standards below depending on how content is assigned.

MIDDLE SCHOOL STANDARDS TARGETS

Structures & Processes

MS-LS1-1. Conduct an investigation to provide evidence that living things are made of cells; either one cell or many different numbers and types of cells.

MS-LS1-3. Use argument supported by evidence for how the body is a system of interacting subsystems composed of groups of cells.

HIGH SCHOOL STANDARDS TARGETS

Structure & Function

HS-LS1-1. Construct an explanation based on evidence for how the structure of DNA determines the structure of proteins which carry out the essential functions of life through systems of specialized cells.

HS-LS1-2. Develop and use a model to illustrate the hierarchical organization of interacting systems that provide specific functions within multicellular organisms.

Matter & Energy in Organisms & Ecosystems

HS-LS1-7. Use a model to illustrate that cellular respiration is a chemical process whereby the bonds of food molecules and oxygen molecules are broken and the bonds in new compounds are formed, resulting in a net transfer of energy.

Inheritance & Variation of Traits

HS-LS3-3. Apply concepts of statistics and probability to explain the variation and distribution of expressed traits in a population.

Natural Selection & Evolution

HS-LS4-1. Communicate scientific information that common ancestry and biological evolution are supported by multiple lines of empirical evidence.

CPSIA information can be obtained
at www.ICGtesting.com
Printed in the USA
JSHW060335120723
44603JS00008B/62

9 781792 422164